Praise for *Travelers to Unimaginable Lands*

A BBC book of the week
A *Telegraph* best book for summer 2023
A *Guardian* best book of 2023

"A book so humane and quietly profound that everyone should read it."

—*Financial Times*

"[Dasha] Kiper's work is deeply moving and often surprising. Through case studies both tragic and hauntingly relatable, she provides scientific grounding for what the beleaguered caregivers go through. With understanding comes the permission for, and perhaps a chance at, self-forgiveness."

—*The Wall Street Journal*

"[One of] the best of this year's books about dementia . . . Invoke[s] literature, art, and pop culture to help explain what science and medicine, in all their lab-coated well-meaningness, cannot fully."

—*The New York Times*

"Kiper . . . evinces a capaciousness of sympathy and understanding for Alzheimer's patients and (especially) their caregivers. . . . For the frustrated caregiver, trapped in a vicious psychodynamic that is dehumanizing to both parties, this may provide some valuable solace."

—*The American Scholar*

T0112873

"An elegant, empathetic, immensely informative, and insightful primer for caregivers as they try to navigate the fragmented, skewed world of the cognitively impaired."
—*Psychology Today*

"A work of exceptional compassion . . . deeply imaginative . . . immeasurably valuable."
—*The Guardian*

"This book will forever change the way we see people with dementia disorders—and the people who care for them. Kiper compassionately illuminates the complex bond between us and our loved ones suffering from cognitive decline, surprising us with what we can learn about ourselves through this experience and the ways our own minds both deceive us and make us uniquely human."
—LORI GOTTLIEB,
New York Times bestselling author of
Maybe You Should Talk to Someone

"Kiper can write with a Sacks-like clarity. . . . A wise book, and one that is unsettling in the best way."
—*New Scientist*

"What if caregivers are just as much victims of Alzheimer's as their charges? . . . A fascinating account of the psychology of caregiving . . . The message of this compassionate book is that confusion is, deep down, part of the human condition."
—*The Daily Telegraph*

"A kind and thought-provoking book, poignant and full of rich insights from neuroscience and social psychology, skillfully introduced to make the stories come alive . . . Dasha Kiper's book is full of accessible insights into the complexity of traveling between past, present, and future, and her rich and humane perspective is hopeful as well as grounded in the reality of what people suffer."

—GWEN ADSHEAD,
author of *The Devil You Know*

"Fascinating . . . a worthwhile and accessible read both for carers and those who may not understand the pressures under which these often underappreciated workers must somehow find ways to survive the loss of a loved one who continues to live."

—*Bookmunch*

"A humane approach to the silent epidemic of cognitive decline."

—*Kirkus Reviews*

"In this thoughtful debut, Kiper, a clinical supervisor at an Alzheimer's caregiving organization, digs into the tortuous effects of dementia for sufferers and caregivers alike. . . . Those dealing with dementia will find solace in this compassionate investigation of the human mind."

—*Publishers Weekly*

"Filled with insights and clinical jewels from start to finish, this book has much to teach us about the brain, our emotions, and the self. It is a treasure."

—NORMAN DOIDGE,
author of *The Brain That Changes Itself*

Travelers to Unimaginable Lands

Travelers
to
Unimaginable
Lands

Stories of
Dementia,
the Caregiver,
and the
Human Brain

Dasha Kiper

RANDOM HOUSE
NEW YORK

2024 Random House Trade Paperback Edition

Copyright © 2023 by Dasha Kiper

Foreword copyright © 2023 by Norman Doidge

All rights reserved.

Published in the United States by Random House, an imprint and division of Penguin Random House LLC, New York.

RANDOM HOUSE and the HOUSE colophon are registered trademarks of Penguin Random House LLC.

Originally published in hardcover in slightly different form in the United States by Random House, an imprint and division of Penguin Random House LLC, in 2023.

Library of Congress Cataloging-in-Publication Data

Names: Kiper, Dasha, author.

Title: Travelers to unimaginable lands: stories of dementia, the caregiver, and the human brain / Dasha Kiper.

Description: New York: Random House, [2022] | Includes bibliographical references and index.

Identifiers: LCCN 2023001949 (print) | LCCN 2023001950 (ebook) | ISBN 9780399590559 | ISBN 9780399590542 (ebook)

Subjects: LCSH: Dementia—Patients—Family relationships—United States. | Dementia—Patients—Care—United States. | Caregivers—Mental health—United States.

Classification: LCC RC521 .K574 2022 (print) | LCC RC521 (ebook) | DDC 362.1968/31—dc23/eng/20230414

LC record available at lccn.loc.gov/2023001949

LC ebook record available at lccn.loc.gov/2023001950

Printed in the United States of America on acid-free paper

randomhousebooks.com

1 2 3 4 5 6 7 8 9

Book design by Susan Turner

To my parents, Masha (Mariya) and Alex Kiper

Foreword

Norman Doidge

TRAVELERS TO UNIMAGINABLE LANDS IS THAT RARITY: TRUE BIBLIO-therapy. Lucid, mature, wise, with hardly a wasted word, it not only deepens our understanding of what transpires as we care for a loved one with Alzheimer's, it also has the potential to be powerfully therapeutic, offering the kind of support and reorientation so essential to the millions of people struggling with the long, often agonizing leave-taking of loved ones stricken with the dreaded disease. The book is based on a profound insight: the concept of "dementia blindness," which identifies a singular problem of caring for people with dementia disorders—one that has generally escaped notice but, once understood, may make a significant difference for many caregivers.

Elegantly written and accessible, *Travelers* is full of frank, lively, and illuminating conversations between the author, Dasha Kiper, and caregivers, which explore the ways caregivers get stuck in patterns hard to escape. These conversations—each of which come from actual clinical encounters—are buttressed by the relevant brain science and interspersed with apt observations drawn from great literature (Borges, Kafka, Chekhov, Melville, Sartre, Beckett) that illuminate the conundrums the disease presents. The topic may be heavy, but the author writes with great sensitivity and a light touch.

Travelers is sorely needed, for several reasons. As of this moment, none of the mainstream drugs for dementia disorders does much to reverse cognitive decline, except to offer a few months of lessening symptoms. When it comes to the treatment of people with Alzheimer's, all the promissory notes of medical science, and the monthly hype about a single magic bullet that will cure this disease, clash with real-world medicine. Indeed, it is becoming increasingly clear that the amyloid hypothesis upon which so many of these claims have been based—the idea that Alzheimer's is caused by nothing but the buildup of plaque in the brain—is woefully inadequate to explain the disease.

In the meantime, it is up to family members and friends, where possible, to take care of their loved ones for much of the duration of their cognitive and physical decline. And yet there has been far too little clinical attention paid to the caregivers themselves. How can we help them through a process that is profoundly difficult, if not traumatic? Remember, alongside the rigors of providing day-to-day care, the caregivers often suffer from what might best be called "anticipatory grief," as familiar aspects of their loved ones slip away. And this may be compounded by a fear, in family members, that they might inherit the disease unfolding in front of them.

Kiper's core insight concerns a counterintuitive dynamic that often occurs between patients and caregivers—a dynamic that has eluded so many, probably because it requires the right person immersing herself in a situation most people wish to avoid. Kiper herself is one of a small cadre who have made it their vocation to help care for the caregivers. She is also a writer with the keenest of minds, combining therapeutic tact and brutal honesty, not only about the process of caregiving but also about her own errors, from which she steadily learns.

Alzheimer's has different presentations and takes a different course in each patient, depending, in part, on where the process begins in the brain. That said, it's often noted that Alzheimer's interferes with short-term memory, leads to other deficits, includes a lot of denial, and, ultimately, leads many victims to gradually "lose their minds."

The genius of this book is to show more precisely the process of resisting such losses as it unfolds *between* patient and caregiver, affecting not just one but both. To learn about this process is surprisingly helpful—not curative, but helpful.

Travelers to Unimaginable Lands clarifies why we, the caregivers, often behave like Sisyphus of the Greek myth, doomed eternally to roll a boulder up a hill, only to watch it roll down again. In similar fashion, we find ourselves repeating the same errors, making the same requests, and getting pulled into the same power struggles, pointless quarrels, and seething ambivalences as we care for our patients. This is partly because Alzheimer's patients seem unable to learn from their mistakes. But it is also because, weirdly enough, caregivers experience the same problem. In an uncanny mirroring, we get pulled into a parallel process with our charges, forgetting what happened yesterday, repeating what didn't work last time, becoming ever more prone to agitation and impatience, even as we're engaged in a trial of devotion that pushes love to its limit.

Why does this happen? Precisely because, as Kiper shows, the healthy brain has evolved to automatically attribute to other people the existence of a self that is sustained over time, has self-reflective capacities, and is capable of learning and absorbing new information. This attribution is the brain's unconscious default position, or cognitive-emotional bias, and does not simply disappear when we become caregivers for people whose own brains begin to falter. It is the invisible projection upon which each human encounter begins, a projection that is implicit in our every conversation and even in the structure of human language itself.

When we say "you," we believe we're talking to another "self," an essence, or perhaps process, that somehow persists over time. But this self—and the continuity it implies—depends on having the memory capacity to knit together our different mental states. This same capacity contributes to the ability to self-reflect, which is a key component of human consciousness. Alzheimer's and related dementia disorders silently strip their victims of the cognitive infrastructure that helps construct this self.

The "loss of self" described in the Alzheimer's literature can happen slowly—over a decade in some cases—and may be stealthy enough that neither the victim (and this is the key point) *nor* the caregiver appreciates its full extent. Alzheimer's notwithstanding, the person remains in front of us, in their usual form and appearance, exhibiting the same expressions, carrying the same music in their voices, evoking in us thousands of familiar memories and emotional associations. There are better and worse days, and sometimes the old self seems to return, with strong will intact—a viable simulacrum of who they once were. Clearly, there is a person there.

Yet as the disease advances, we may come to see just the shell or the husk of the self we once knew. But this new understanding does not stop us from projecting a continuous self, because, as Kiper explains, it is the brain's default position—that is, we cannot help but see what was once there. This brilliant insight is the entry point into the hitherto difficult to imagine land she goes on to describe.

We often say of people caught in this bind—knowing the loved one's self is diminished but continuing to see it as whole—that they are "in denial," as if this was only a defense mechanism at work. But that is a misapplication of the valuable term "denial." Yes, there can be denial, and Kiper describes some of it. But those caught in the Sisyphean entanglement are not simply denying that their loved ones are ill—after all, they're the ones accepting infirmity and trying to help. Though it may accompany denial or even reinforce it, dementia blindness isn't simply the defense mechanism of a stressed mind; it is, as Kiper shows, a product of how the healthy mind normally works. This is one reason why the discovery of the concept has been so elusive, and why this book is so helpful.

Until now, we have been forced to cobble together our

picture of what it is like to have Alzheimer's subjectively. We have had no perfect guide. After all, there has never been a case of someone reversing the process in its very advanced stage (after the self has been radically diminished) and returning to share what it was like and how best to relate to people in extremis. So there has always been something imprecise and necessarily provisional when we use such haunting phrases as "loss of self." At the same time, there has also been a tendency to not take seriously enough what might be the second-best form of guidance: the firsthand observations of professional caregivers. This is because they are all too often relegated to the lower rungs of the healthcare hierarchy by a medical system, and a zeitgeist, that often only looks up to and listens to those who promise "cures," thinking nothing less will do.

DASHA KIPER IS A PERCEPTIVE observer who stays close to her material. But as sometimes happens when an observer is meticulous in describing a particular experience, a more general insight can emerge. Although Kiper makes no such claims, it is entirely possible that her approach, which shows how the cognitive biases of both the patient and the caregiver interlock, may be of assistance in thinking about other kinds of brain-based problems that affect aspects of the self and its continuity over time.

To take one example: schizophrenia. When it was first diagnosed in 1883, it was called "dementia praecox," because doctors believed that a patient's brain was prematurely deteriorating. When most of us think of schizophrenia, however, we tend to associate the illness with its more prominent symptoms, like hallucinations and delusions. But, in fact, there are often other less prominent or "noisy" symptoms, like cognitive decline; hence the original name. As with dementia disorders, such changes to the infrastructure of the self may not be detected by the patient themselves or seen clearly by the caregiver.

People caring for those afflicted with schizophrenia may have trouble seeing the extent to which the disease has altered their loved ones. Again, this is usually written off as denial. But while denial may be operative, we have to wonder, given Kiper's insights, if this particular blind spot is not also a product of the workings of the caregiver's mind projecting onto their loved one, by default, the same experience of self they had before the onset of the illness. This is not to say schizophrenia is the same as Alzheimer's. Of course it's not, and, thankfully it has a better prognosis and better treatment. But Kiper's insight into the causes of dementia blindness may be relevant, in modified form, to this and other neurological and psychiatric conditions.

For practical purposes, an awareness of dementia blindness may help caregivers bypass some cognitive roadblocks, allowing them to better empathize with the person suffering from the disease and even disengage from unproductive entanglements.

I have used the word "person" here, as distinguished from "self," because, as I read it, the thrust of this book is to be respectful of the dignity of the person. Far from using the insight into loss of self as a way to dehumanize the patient, *Travelers to Unimaginable Lands* aspires to a more humane approach to the patient's cognitive state, in which the diminishment of self may be disguised by the caregiver's own biases and intuitions.

If I seem to be struggling with what term ("person," "self," "patient") best describes people with serious cognitive decline, it's because Kiper's work opens up new territory for which we don't yet have proper vocabulary or concepts—be they psychological, neurological, legal, or colloquial—that can help us to think about people who progressively evince a lack of continuity of self. No doubt, this absence of vocabulary has made it hard to think through the implications of dementia blindness in society at large. But, in the meantime, more important than finding the right word is finding the right guide, a person willing and able to take us into (if not completely through) this often unimaginable land—someone who knows its strangeness and its pitfalls.

A wise old medical adage, apt for real-world medicine, is this: "To cure sometimes, to relieve often, to comfort always." I believe this book may well relieve and comfort, by clarifying the caregiver-patient relationship for many a tormented, confused, guilt-laden, self-attacking caregiver. Alzheimer's, like any other kind of serious disease, reminds us of our own mortality, while also stirring up many unresolved issues with the person we are caring for. Kiper's psychologically astute observations deepen our understanding of why so many difficult encounters occur between caregiver and patient, why they cause us pain, and what might beneficially be gleaned from them.

Which brings me to one last counterintuitive point. The experience of reading Dasha Kiper's book may not be quite what one expects. Perusing its pages is not only grounding and often touching, it is sometimes even uplifting, as we meet people facing head-on something that looms large for so many of us. Kiper lets us accompany caregivers as they struggle to accept, acknowledge, cope with, and ultimately survive the loss of someone they love. Filled with insights and clinical jewels from start to finish, this book has much to teach us about the brain, our emotions, and the self. It is a treasure.

NORMAN DOIDGE, M.D., is the author of *The Brain That Changes Itself* and *The Brain's Way of Healing*.

Contents

WHEN I WAS TWENTY-FIVE YEARS OLD, I MOVED IN WITH A MAN who was ninety-eight. I had not planned to, I wasn't sure I wanted to, and I didn't know if I could do any good. This man, whom I'll call Mr. Kessler, wasn't a friend or relative. He was a Holocaust survivor in the first stages of Alzheimer's disease, and I'd been hired to look after him. Although I had a background in clinical psychology, I was by no means a professional caregiver. I was hired because Mr. Kessler's son, Sam, thought his father shouldn't live alone—not necessarily because he was unfit, but because he could use some help around the house.

Like many victims of Alzheimer's, Mr. Kessler did not acknowledge his condition and went about life as though burdened by the normal aches and pains of aging rather than by an irrevocable and debilitating disease. If he put the laundry detergent in the oven or forgot which floor he lived on, he'd shake his head and sigh, *"Mayn kop arbet nisht"* ("My head doesn't work"). But it was a lament, not a diagnosis. And this denial, both clinical and profoundly human, led his son to misjudge the illness as well.

Once ensconced in Mr. Kessler's two-bedroom apartment in the Bronx, I became, as so many caregivers do, a record keeper of someone else's obsessions: "Where are my keys?" "Have you seen my wallet?" "What day is it?" "Where do you live?" "Where do your parents live?" He didn't ask these questions every day in the year I cared for him, he asked them nine or ten times a day, every day. And since he always asked them for the "first" time, his sense of urgency never waned and that urgency became my own. I wanted to help him, but I couldn't. I wanted him to appreciate my efforts, but *he* couldn't.

A year before I moved in, in 2009, I was on an academic track to get a Ph.D. in clinical psychology, studying pathology primarily through the dispassionate lens of quantitative analysis, with an emphasis on depression, PTSD, complicated grief, and anxiety. Although in some ways my studies were rewarding, I felt alienated by the generalities of research and the sterile, impersonal study of illness. I understood that empirical data and clinical trials were essential, but I also knew they did not offer a complete perspective on neurological illness, and I soon became disillusioned with dogmas and theoretical frameworks.

What ultimately drew me away from academia is the same thing that initially drew me to it: Before I was a student of clinical psychology, I was a student of Dr. Oliver Sacks. I never met Dr. Sacks, but since I had first picked up *The Man Who Mistook His Wife for a Hat* as a teenager, I had internalized his voice, his sensibility, his frame of reference. What made me fall for Dr. Sacks was how much he fell for his patients. As he narrated their stories, seamlessly integrating neurology with the study of identity, it became impossible to tease apart his clinical observations from his affection. Perhaps that's why I loved that he adopted the term "romantic science" from his friend and mentor Alexander Luria, a Soviet neuropsychologist, to describe his work.

Although the term "romantic science" is a nod to the eighteenth-century tradition of incorporating personal details into the study of illness, it also felt fitting in the more vernacular sense. Dr. Sacks was so deeply moved and impressed by how his patients navigated their worlds and built meaning into their lives, both despite and because of their conditions, that his case studies seemed not just explorations of human consciousness but also odes to individual human beings. So when I was asked to look after Mr. Kessler, I saw it as an opportunity to observe how a person fights to preserve his sense of self even as a neurological disease was eroding it.

Some mornings Mr. Kessler knew who I was; some mornings he did not. Some days he resented my presence; some days he was glad to have my company. And some days, as if in gentle reproof to his own forgetfulness, he looked at me and murmured, "How long have I been like this?" Or "Why don't I remember?" Or "I don't know how you put up with me." Although this shuttling between confusion and self-awareness is often part of the disease, it is not typically reflected in clinical discourse. Instead, we have words like "insight" to address the knowledge patients supposedly have about their condition. But such words strike me as naïvely binary. Insight isn't a switch that turns on or off in someone with dementia. Indeed, no description of a patient's awareness can capture the complex, contradictory nature of a mind under duress, or, for that matter, of the mind that seeks to alleviate such duress.

For his part, Oliver Sacks disliked the term "deficit," which he considered "neurology's favorite word." He disliked it because it tends to reduce the patient to a functional system that either works or doesn't work. As with "insight," the term doesn't allow for ambiguity. And what is both poignant and unnerving about dementia disorders—which are presumably all about deficit: loss of memory, loss of attention, loss of inhibition, loss of judgment—is that before such loss occurs, there is often abundance—an abundance of yelling, arguing, defending, fabricating, and accusing. More to the point, there is often an abundance of the self. Where there is loss, there may be compensating behaviors, moments when the brain does not surrender to the disease but arms itself with those faculties that are still intact, marshaling everything it can to compensate for what is slipping away.

We refer to this kind of compensation as leaning on our "cognitive reserve," which is both apt and ironic given the upheaval and chaos this hidden resource creates for patient and caregiver. By using the networks that still function, the brain tries to preserve a person's sense of self, enabling patients to argue, charm, convince, fabricate, accuse, and persist.* All of which makes the line between pathology and

---

* Throughout this book I use "mind" and "brain" interchangeably, but I favor "the brain" when describing specific processes and "the mind" when speaking generally about human nature. My usage does not signal an endorsement of either side of the complex and heated "mind-body" debate.

resilience increasingly murky. Indeed, we might say it's a patient's cognitive reserve rather than dementia disorders that initially accounts for the behavior that bedevils us.

Unlike cancer or congestive heart failure, diseases of the brain present no demarcation between the illness and the patient. Patients "collude" with their malady and become, as Dr. Sacks put it, "a long-married couple . . . a single compound being." In which case, who exactly is responsible for odd or contrary behavior? The man who charged into my bedroom in the middle of the night and asked me to find his passport was also the man who told me two minutes after I located it to get out because he had no need for me. The man who quietly spoke to me for hours about his childhood was also the man who told his son that he and I never interacted and that he'd prefer to live alone.

The more I came to know Mr. Kessler, the more I saw him as a "compound" being whose contradictions were not merely a by-product of cognitive decline but manifestations of a man who wanted it both ways: to be completely independent and yet receive constant attention. And it was *that* man in collusion with the disease that kept me off balance. Ironically, the very quality I admired in Dr. Sacks's patients, "the preservation of the self," was now making my job much more difficult.

As Mr. Kessler teetered between knowing and not knowing me, between wanting my company and rejecting it, between happily eating the meals I prepared and accusing me of taking advantage of his hospitality, I felt myself pulled between feeling useful and feeling like an intruder. His oscillations began to tug at my own sense of existential rootlessness. Why was I here? What was I doing? Was I doing any good at all? It was my first indication that people with dementia disorders can still find your most vulnerable part and poke at it until you yourself feel unraveled.

One evening, about seven months into my stay, Mr. Kessler haltingly climbed on top of a chair to change the battery in a smoke detector. When I warned him how dangerous this was and offered to help, he snapped, in typical fashion, that he was the boss and didn't need help. Usually, when he tried to fix things, I would distract him. But this time, for just one minute, I needed him to understand that there was such a thing as objective reality. "Forget about the alarm," I said firmly. "It's too dangerous." He waved me away and put a foot on the chair. Aggravated by his condescension, I felt an uncharacteristic urge to strip him of his delusions. I was tired of playing this game, tired of being his co-conspirator in the belief that nothing was wrong with him, which, ironically, made it easier for him to question my presence in his home. So I did what caregivers shouldn't: I argued. Shaking with indignation, I shouted that he didn't do anything by himself, that he always needed my help, that he wasn't capable of living alone.

Although my outburst didn't seem to faze him and fled his memory after ten minutes, it so disturbed me that for weeks I succumbed to apathy. I'd still perform my usual tasks—feeding Mr. Kessler the lines he wanted to hear, prompting him to tell his stories, reminding him of the people who had called that day—but I often felt hopeless and numb. Moreover, I thought I was failing, perhaps not in my duties, but as a human being. What did it say about me that

I could yell at a ninety-nine-year-old man suffering from dementia? Where was the "compassionate detachment" Dr. Sacks deemed indispensable for looking after the neurologically impaired? The doctor, of course, could leave his patients at the end of the day and return to his house in the West Village to relax and recharge. I, on the other hand, had nowhere to go. Even so, I felt I was betraying what I had learned from his books.

It was only right, then, that one of his books should come to my rescue. One day, glancing through *The Man Who Mistook His Wife for a Hat,* I was struck by a paragraph that I had probably read a dozen times before. It appears in the case of "The Lost Mariner," which deals with a "charming, intelligent, memoryless" man who lived in New York City's Home for the Aged. "Jimmie R.," as Dr. Sacks called him, suffered from Korsakoff syndrome, which left him unable to form new memories. As a result, he believed himself nineteen years old when, in fact, he was forty-nine. Perhaps because the contrast between Jimmie R.'s self-image and his reality was so stark, Dr. Sacks gave in to a sudden impulse: He held a mirror up to his face and told him to look. Jimmie R. was naturally horrified and panic-stricken by what he saw. Immediately realizing his mistake, Dr. Sacks soothed Jimmie until he forgot what the mirror had shown him. But Dr. Sacks didn't forget and never forgave himself for what he had done.

Reading that passage, I felt grateful to him. Grateful that he had made a mistake and had the grace to acknowledge it. Grateful that he let us know that he was a flawed human being who for a moment had behaved irrationally. Why had he put a mirror in front of a patient who could not abide the truth? Even Dr. Sacks, it seems, felt the same compulsion that many caregivers feel. Does not every caregiver sooner or later hold a mirror up to their loved one? Don't all of us plead and try to reason with patients in order to make them grasp what's real and what isn't? Like any caregiver, Dr. Sacks instinctively wanted to fix his patient, to make him normal again. It's the reason we argue with and sometimes yell at our charges; we want to reestablish a shared reality. It's not cruelty but desperation that drives us to confront them with the truth.

My perspective began to shift: "The Lost Mariner" was not just about someone who endured the "continuing pressure of anomaly and contradiction," vainly seeking continuity while "stuck in a constantly changing, meaningless moment." It was also about Dr. Sacks and all the caregivers who find themselves sucked into that meaningless moment with the cognitively impaired.

THE WORD "DEMENTIA," FROM THE Latin *de* (deprived of or out of) + *mens* (mind), entered the English lexicon in the late eighteenth century and originally denoted madness or insanity. As medicine belatedly began to address disorders of the mind as well as those of the body, signs of befuddlement, senility, and personality change began to be viewed in a somatic light and finally in the last century as neurological issues. *The Diagnostic and Statistical Manual of Mental Disorders,* fifth edition (*DSM-5*), has, in fact, discouraged the use of the term "dementia," opting instead for "neurological disorders." This shift to the biological has helped to destigmatize behaviors that were once considered shameful. Would you get angry at someone who has cancer or heart disease?

Although "dementia" is still commonly used to identify an illness, the term, in fact, simply covers a cluster of different symptoms associated with cognitive decline, such as memory loss, poor emotional control, and difficulty with judgment, planning, and problem-solving. Dementia can be temporary and is occasionally caused by drugs, dehydration, or a vitamin deficiency, but dementia disorders such as Alzheimer's disease, Lewy body dementia, frontotemporal dementia, and vascular dementia are diseases, and they are irreversible.

More than fifty-five million people live with a dementia disorder worldwide, and by 2050 that number is expected to almost triple. Alzheimer's disease is the most common type of dementia, and some 6.5 million people in America exhibit symptoms ranging from mild cognitive impairment to full-blown Alzheimer's. Although aging is the strongest risk factor, dementia does not exclusively affect the elderly; early onset dementias (where symptoms appear before the age of sixty-five) account for up to 9 percent of cases. The global cost of treating these disorders is estimated to be $1.3 trillion a year and will more than double in ten years.

Looking after the afflicted in the United States are well over eleven million caregivers (the number worldwide is too large to venture a guess), many of whom are family members who annually provide over $271 billion worth of unpaid care. Perhaps more significant is the staggering physical and psychological cost to their own health as a result of caregiving. It is these individuals who have been dubbed the "invisible victims" of the disease. Yet even this small gesture of recognition does not reflect the truer and darker meaning of "victim."

Dementia disorders, in many cases, create a world so fragmented, so skewed, so redundant, so indifferent to normal rules of behavior that family members unwittingly become part of the madness. Yet clinicians and researchers continue to posit a clear distinction between the mind of the caregiver and that of the patient, between the normal and the abnormal, when, in fact, the true burden for caregivers is often the absence of such a divide.* Children and spouses do not merely witness their loved one's cognitive decline, they become part of it, living in its surreal, bleak reality every minute of every day.

I read a lot about dementia disorders during and after my days in the Bronx. I read the medical literature. I read memoirs of caregivers describing the emotional toll the disease takes. I pored over scholarly articles about the social, economic, and logistical problems that arise when these diseases invade a family setting. I consulted practical guidebooks offering advice on how to manage, cope with, and communicate effectively with those afflicted. But as informative and supportive as such books are, as accurately as they portray the effects of the disease, I still felt something was missing from the conversation.

Although we expect irrational behavior and lapses of judgment from Alzheimer's patients, we're often puzzled by

---

* I use the term "patient" as a shorthand so as not to say "person with dementia." Such usage in no way changes the status of anyone being cared for by someone other than a medical professional. Nor should it suggest that cognitive impairment defines a person's selfhood.

the baffling behavior of caregivers themselves, many of whom mirror the denial, resistance, distortions, irrationality, and cognitive lapses of the people they're caring for. Indeed, caregivers, despite recognizing that their charges are ill, find themselves engaging in behaviors they know are counterproductive: arguing, blaming, insisting on reality, and taking symptoms personally. Because caregivers are "healthy," we assume they should be reasonable, which is what makes their inability to accept or adapt to the disease feel like a personal shortcoming.

Traditionally, neurological case studies have focused on the "abnormal" brain and its effects on the patient. But what about the people closest to the patient? Might not *their* reactions, *their* struggles, *their* own disorientation in the face of neurological illness also illuminate the workings of the human mind? The "normal" mind, after all, is not just a blank slate, or tabula rasa, as John Locke suggested. We now know it is riddled with instincts, drives, needs, and intuitions about ourselves and others. It is these very cognitive proclivities, as I will reveal, that get in the way of understanding and dealing with dementia.

When someone's memory disappears, when personality and behavior change, whom then are we dealing with? When a neurological disease affects the brain, how do our expectations of people change? When is it right to treat them differently? Suddenly, questions usually aired by philosophers and psychologists—about identity, free will, consciousness, memory, and the mind-body connection—make their way into the daily lives of caregivers.

And this is what I would like to explore: How the healthy

brain's cognitive biases and philosophical intuitions affect our understanding and treatment of people who can no longer care for themselves. My case studies are therefore always about two people—patient and caregiver—who unknowingly collaborate in misinterpreting the disease. Relying on cognitive and neurological research as well as on my own experience, I want to show how both patient and caregiver react to the existential dilemma created by dementia. For it is by examining how both grapple with the disease that we catch a fresh glimpse into the hidden workings of the mind.

FOURTEEN MONTHS AFTER I MOVED to the Bronx, I left Mr. Kessler in the care of full-time aides provided by a city agency. Still unsure about graduate school, I moved back to Manhattan and trained to become a group leader for those experiencing the emotional hardships of caring for family members. Such groups provide a safe haven where caregivers can share their thoughts and struggles, knowing they'll be understood by people living through similar situations. In time I became the Consulting Clinical Director of Support Groups for an Alzheimer's organization, responsible for the training and supervision of group leaders, while also continuing to lead groups myself.*

The longer I'm in this field and the more I learn from caregivers, the more I'm convinced that the "healthy" brain

---

* To ensure the anonymity and privacy of the people I have spoken to, I have changed the names, identifying details, and in some cases the dates that appear in the following case studies.

did not evolve to accommodate dementia disorders. As one caregiver aptly put it to me: "Being a caregiver is like being an anthropologist on Mars." She was referring to Oliver Sacks's famous case study in which a woman with autism, Temple Grandin, described herself as an anthropologist because what came easily, even unconsciously, to other people was alien to her. She had to study and learn behaviors that were instinctive for others. Caregivers also find themselves on Mars, but their problem is reversed. Dementia disorders create an environment in which our social instincts are no longer useful—in fact, they're counterproductive. All the misunderstandings, arguments, and recriminations between caregivers and patients point to a problem our brains are not equipped to solve: The unconscious biases and assumptions we've always relied on now lead us astray.

It is no simple matter to live with a person who blatantly disregards the rules of time, order, and continuity. So instead of offering platitudes or redemptive lessons, I want to normalize the caregiver's denial, anger, frustration, and helplessness by explaining why miscommunications occur. This, I hope, will validate their struggles and remove the stigma of failing to live up to an impossible ideal.

Because patients compensate for as long as they can, caregivers witness not only the disease but also the person pushing back against the disease. We might assume that acknowledging a patient's humanity makes us better caregivers, and of course this is true. We should never lose sight of the fact that we're dealing with human beings who have thoughts and feelings. But it is also true that in long-standing relationships, acknowledging the humanity of someone with a dementia disorder complicates our feelings and makes it hard not to take their symptoms personally. So we must learn to understand not only the man who mistakes his wife for a hat but also the wife who must adapt to a husband who mistakes her for a hat.

These days, as I walk home in the evenings after seeing caregivers, I think about what they've told me. I try to imagine their lives, the problems they face, and the adjustments they have to make day by day and hour by hour. And I call to mind Dr. Sacks's description of patients who are "travelers to unimaginable lands—lands of which otherwise we should have no idea or conception." And I want to chime in: "Let's not forget about the caregivers who must travel with them." Because once you hear the stories that caregivers have to tell, once you learn about their sorrows and struggles and their resolve to endure, you, too, may see them—or yourself—in the same sympathetic light that Dr. Sacks shines on his wards: as archetypal figures of classical fable, "heroes, victims, martyrs, warriors."

Travelers to Unimaginable Lands

1

Borges in the Bronx

Why We Can't Remember That
Alzheimer's Patients Forget

*One day in 1887, a young man saddles his horse and goes out
riding. Perhaps the horse is spooked or stumbles, and the young
man is thrown hard to the ground. He loses consciousness, and
when he recovers he learns that he is hopelessly crippled. He
retires to his modest ranch in southwestern Uruguay, where he
is visited one night by a writer of his acquaintance. The writer
finds him lying on a cot, immersed in darkness, smoking a cigarette and reciting in a high-pitched voice the words of a Latin
treatise. After an exchange of pleasantries, the young man,
whose name is Ireneo Funes, brings up another outcome of his
accident. It seems he now possesses an imperishable memory.
Everything from an object's form to its shadow, every experience*

and how he feels about it, is filed away precisely as it occurs. He can recall not only "every leaf on every tree of every wood, but even every one of the times he had perceived or imagined it." He can learn any language in a matter of hours, reconstruct all of his dreams, and has in fact reconstructed an entire day, minute by tumultuous minute. "I have more memories in myself alone than all men have had since the world was a world," he tells the writer.

The two men talk through the night, and when the sun rises, the writer, for the first time, makes out Funes's face. He seems "more ancient than Egypt, older than the prophecies and the pyramids." And suddenly the writer realizes the cost of owning an implacable memory, a memory that never allows us to forget, a memory that calls into question the very purpose of remembering.

TO GET TO MR. KESSLER'S neighborhood in the Bronx from Columbia University, you take the 1 train to 231st Street and transfer to a bus. The trip takes about forty minutes, enough time for me to wonder, on my first ride uptown, whether I'd made a mistake. Had I really left graduate school to look after a ninety-eight-year-old man? I told myself I was a temporary fix, someone to help Mr. Kessler around the house until his son, Sam, found a more permanent solution. But as the weeks wore on and Mr. Kessler's equilibrium was jarred time and again by confusion and emotional outbursts, I became increasingly invested in his struggle. His swings from clear-headedness to bewilderment, sometimes within minutes, made me wonder why caregivers like Sam find profound memory loss so hard to acknowledge, much less accept.

Sam's relationship with his father had been fractious from the time he had announced, at twenty-one, that he was going to be a professional musician. He had picked up a saxophone at twelve and discovered he loved the sound it made. He prevailed upon his father to buy him one and taught himself to play by listening to records and hanging out with other young musicians. Mr. Kessler didn't mind Sam "making noise" in the house, but playing music was no way of making a living. Sam needed to get a job first and play music second. But Sam had no interest in working. His job, he told his father, was playing the tenor sax. "What kind of job is that?" Mr. Kessler had retorted. "You need to work in an office. Be an adult. Adults don't sleep in the day and stay up all night."

But Sam did stay up most nights. He joined various bands, playing in one nightspot after another, making just enough money to get by. When Sam tried to explain what jazz meant to him, Mr. Kessler would shake his head and mutter, "Words, words." What worried him was that Sam's life was unstructured, his career uncertain, and that he had never married.

A Holocaust survivor, Mr. Kessler was a curious mixture of certainty and vulnerability, of innocence and obstinacy. He behaved as if he knew everything, perhaps because everything he had once known had been so brutally snatched away. Perhaps, too, this is why many survivors became overinvested in their children. For them, having children was a kind of vindication, a form of resistance against the Nazis. Although this was never alluded to by Mr. Kessler, it might partly explain why he wanted more than anything else that Sam should lead what Mr. Kessler considered a normal life, a life that could not be upended as his had been.

It was this oppressive concern, as Sam one day confided, that made him attend college out of state and immerse himself so completely in his music. But he could not escape. Not fully. Mr. Kessler's conviction that Sam was wasting his life was relentless. But even as Sam felt burdened by his father's expectations, he also wanted his approval. And though he hated causing him more pain, he also resented being made to feel like a disappointment. But how could he make his father understand this? One believed in rules, the other questioned them; one took refuge in platitudes and convention, the other felt stifled by them. As a result, Mr. Kessler could show love and concern only by urging caution and finding fault, while Sam could protect himself only by pushing against his father's limited worldview.

GIVEN THE BODY OF LITERATURE devoted to caregiving, it's surprising how little attention is paid to the uncanny way that dementia often continues or exacerbates a long-standing dynamic. Indeed, one of the cruelest aspects of the disease— one that dementia guidebooks are loath to mention—is that its symptoms often recapitulate a laundry list of mutually aggravating behaviors. Although such books duly warn caregivers to expect stubbornness, clinginess, defensiveness, suspicion, incessant anxiety, irrationality, argumentativeness, and blatant denials of reality, they view these behaviors only as symptoms of dementia disorders rather than familiar irritants. They are symptoms, of course, but they may also represent problems that have always plagued a familial relationship.

For Sam, the behaviors that had nettled him when his father was sixty irritated him no less now that his father was almost a hundred. His worst offense, in Sam's eyes, was potentially the most harmful: Mr. Kessler's newfound habit of fiddling with the electric fixtures and lamps. At least once a week, I overheard a version of the following:

> SAM: Stop trying to fix the lamp in your room. It's dangerous.
> MR. KESSLER: I don't touch the lamp. I don't know what you want from me.
> SAM: You mess around with the lamp and the wiring. That's how you cut your hand.
> MR. KESSLER: I never touch the wires. What wires have I touched?
> SAM: Don't argue with me! Just do as I say. It's for your own good.
> MR. KESSLER: When do I argue with you?
> SAM: You always argue with me. You're always giving me trouble!
> MR. KESSLER: No one ever said I give anyone trouble.
> SAM: You're giving me trouble right now!
> MR. KESSLER: How? How am I giving you trouble?
> SAM: You don't listen to me. And if you keep arguing and contradicting me, I'll stop coming to see you.
> MR. KESSLER: (worried) I promise. I promise I will listen to you one hundred percent.

SAM: Okay. Now promise me you'll stop touching the lamp in the bedroom. Repeat it to yourself: "I will not touch the lamp!"

MR. KESSLER: (*indignant*) I never touch the lamp. What lamp?

SAM: Goddammit, stop arguing with me!

MR. KESSLER: When do I ever argue with you?

Each time I heard a different permutation of this argument, I felt a wave of protectiveness toward both father and son. Dementia was punishing them in the same way they had always punished each other. And while Mr. Kessler would quickly forget their arguments, they accumulated in Sam's mind until his frustration and anger boiled over—as did his guilt. And when Sam berated himself for losing his temper, I felt as if I were failing both of them. Although I had grown accustomed to feeling helpless when confronted by Mr. Kessler's distress, I thought that surely I could help Sam.

One day, after another bad fight, I took Sam aside and showed him photographs of the healthy brain and the dementia brain, with the hippocampus pitifully shrunken to half its normal size. Staring at the tinted images, Sam looked appropriately somber, struck by the dimmed regions of the dementia brain. Here was indisputable evidence that his father was no longer the person that Sam had been fighting with for decades. Yet only an hour after Sam viewed these photographs, he and his father were shouting at each other again.

It was a lesson to me. Just as I had mistakenly regarded intimate moments with Mr. Kessler as touchstones of closeness, I mistook Sam's moment of clarity for long-term under-standing. In fact, each time I saw a look of somber realization flash across Sam's face, or caught him tenderly reaching for his father's hand to make up for some harsh words, I felt he had finally achieved a sense of acceptance. But invariably Mr. Kessler would do or say something that provoked another outburst, and the same disbelief welled up inside me. It was as if my conversations with Sam about his father's condition had never taken place. Every day it seemed we were starting from scratch. Who, I sometimes wondered, was suffering more from memory loss, Sam or his father?

But the error was mine, not Sam's. I was ignoring what so many mental health professionals also ignore: the cognitive limits of the healthy brain. Of course, it's only natural to define the "healthy" mind in opposition to the afflicted mind, but in reality what makes caregiving so frustrating is that the distinction between a normally functioning brain and an impaired brain is not always clear-cut: Both can give rise to the same kinds of denials and distortions.

In *The Seven Sins of Memory,* the psychologist Daniel L. Schacter identifies the patterns by which memory errs. Some "sins," like "bias," "misattribution," and "suggestibility," are responsible for distorting memories. Others, such as "tran-sience" and "absent-mindedness," weaken them. Although we're usually not mindful of when we "sin," we do know that we sometimes forget. But what we may be less aware of are the compensatory strategies we use to offset memory loss. When we forget, the mind doesn't just throw in the towel; it gets to work, creating narratives to cover its tracks. This may lead to other errors, but it also gives us something more important: a meaningful framework that orients us as we move through the world.

One of memory's roles is to impose order on the environment, organizing and reorganizing the past to give it a sense of coherence. Daniel Schacter explains that when we retrieve a memory, we're not really shining a spotlight on the past, summoning past events as they actually occurred. Instead, we're reconstructing past experience based on *some* elements of what happened, on a general sense of what *might* have happened, and on our current beliefs and feelings. How is this done? Evidently, experiences get stored in the brain as a series of biochemical changes known as "engrams." Each initial act of encoding, or storing information, is highly selective. As we encode, we unconsciously target information that conforms to previous experience, to knowledge we already possess, and to our state of mind at this particular moment. This is why people may have wildly different perceptions and recollections of the same experience.

Moreover, when we retrieve an experience, we don't merely access engrams as a computer does with a piece of stored information. The cues that trigger memory (smells, moods, sounds, and sights) also influence and change those stored (previously chosen) fragments to create something new. In effect, memory is a collaboration between the past and the present. But this, as Schacter notes, is not something that sits well with us. We intuitively believe in "a one-to-one correspondence" between an event stored in our brain (an engram) and what we remember. And yet this is decidedly not the case. The memory of an event, Schacter writes, "is not simply an activated engram [but] a unique pattern that emerges from the pooled contributions of the cue and the engram"—and this is what produces the autobiographical narratives that explain us to ourselves.

Some of these narratives can be surprisingly resilient even in the face of neurological damage. The "personality knowledge" that forms our self-image is not easily damaged by Alzheimer's and other dementias. What is affected, however, is the ability to update this self-image. So when Sam remarked that Mr. Kessler was eating too much, a common tendency in Alzheimer's patients, Mr. Kessler reflexively replied, "Impossible!," since he considered himself someone who did everything in moderation. If Sam begged him to stop asking the same questions over and over, Mr. Kessler denied doing so, since he still regarded himself as someone who "never bothered anyone." And when Sam asked him not to yell at me, Mr. Kessler immediately became indignant. "Never!" he shouted. "I get along with everyone."

But were these denials the product of Alzheimer's or of memory up to its old tricks? For caregivers such ambiguity is a fact of life because Alzheimer's takes an already imperfect memory and makes it even less reliable, thus making it difficult to distinguish between ordinary memory lapses and those arising from the disease. Yet even as such lapses become more frequent and profound, caregivers still find it difficult to recognize pathology since the patient's impulse to create narratives persists.

Perhaps because Mr. Kessler had endured the loss of his family and home, he needed to form an image of himself as a good man, a man who helped others rather than someone who needed help. This unshakable view of himself as self-sufficient and morally upright gave him a sense of well-being and helped him handle life's vicissitudes. So, when confronted by accusations that he was making things difficult for others, he naturally turned to the convictions and biases that had always served him. Like the rest of us, he was helped along by memory's "egocentric bias," which fastens on events that make us look good and edits those that don't. In the end, the stories we tell ourselves are more compelling, more vivid, and more indestructible than experience itself.

SEEING HOW CAPABLY MR. KESSLER both circumvented and compensated for memory loss brought to mind Jorge Luis Borges's short story "Funes the Memorious," whose titular protagonist remembers absolutely everything. What first appears to be a tremendous cognitive advantage is, in its own way, more crippling than memory loss. Unable to forget, Funes is free of the sins of memory. Although these sins seem like a defect, they are, in fact, adaptative features that help us navigate the world. Precisely because you and I cannot retain all the details of experience, our minds are motivated to sum up experience in terms of values, lessons, and meaning. Funes's perfect memory, however, feels no such urge or urgency. For him the world is just there: Every thought, sight, and sound, every experience, is immediately embedded forever. In a real sense, Funes is enslaved by memory, forced to accumulate facts accurate down to the tiniest detail, endlessly increasing but never taking on shape or form.

Anticipating cognitive psychologists by half a century,

Borges extrapolated something fundamental about the nature of memory: Human memory is not geared for accuracy; it's not a tape recording of events but rather a reconstruction of them that allows us to make sense of the world. So while Mr. Kessler might have lost his ability to remember, he—unlike Funes—could still provide what Dr. Sacks describes as "continuity, a narrative continuity, when memory, and thus experience, [are] being snatched away every instant."

What helps the patient cope, however, may frustrate the caregiver. The more Alzheimer's took away from Mr. Kessler, the more he clung to his self-serving narrative and the more he denied anything that contradicted his self-image. To Sam this denial was not a by-product of a shrinking hippocampus but a sign of his father's typical lack of self-awareness. Of course, Sam's own bias also kept him from recognizing memory loss.

Because memory is biased toward preexisting knowledge, we all "edit" the present to make it look like the past. No matter what new symptoms his father presented, Sam's memory encoded his father's behavior in a way that made him *appear* more consistent with the man he used to know. Thus both patients' and caregivers' biases collaborate to make the disease seem less pervasive than it really is.

Sadly, it's only when patients become truly helpless and unable to compensate that others can see the disease clearly. One night when Sam decided to stay over, he found his father in the hall reaching for the telephone.

"Who are you calling?" Sam asked.

"My son," Mr. Kessler replied.

"Oh?" said Sam. "Who am I?"

"You're Sam," his father said, impervious to the contradiction and chuckling at the silliness of the question. He continued to dial.

For a moment, Sam seemed stunned. He then walked over to his father and gently hung up the phone. The look on his face told me everything I wanted to know. He had finally realized that something was happening that had nothing to do with him. His father had traveled someplace where Sam could not follow, a place that he had to accept if he was going to help his father (and himself) deal with the disease.

This is it, I thought. *He's got it.*

But he hadn't, not fully. Once Mr. Kessler seemed himself again, Sam's insight dimmed and their old dynamic was restored.

AFTER MR. KESSLER DEVELOPED ALZHEIMER'S, father and son exchanged roles. Now it was Sam who did the worrying. Like his father before him, Sam tended to hover, to micromanage, to insist that life be normal. And now it was Mr. Kessler who demanded space, who insisted on his independence, who seemed determined to prove that he knew what he was doing. The intolerance that Mr. Kessler had once exhibited toward Sam was now being visited on him.

Like many adult children, Sam found it hard to see the man he knew slipping away. It seemed unfair, even cruel, that Mr. Kessler, having lost his family in the war and his wife to cancer, should now lose them all over again by having them disappear from memory. So Sam did what he could to help preserve them. When he came to visit, he listened patiently to the same stories he had heard a hundred times before. He took pleasure in his father's reminiscences about the Warsaw he grew up in, surrounded by the people he loved. And it was during those moments, when his father relaxed and let his son care for him, that Sam appeared the happiest.

Just as Alzheimer's can magnify conflict, it can also bring out affection and tenderness: quiet moments when arguments cease, when Mr. Kessler, half asleep, would reach for his son's hand. Perhaps because of an increased desire for comfort or the lowering of inhibitions, or perhaps because tending to a patient's needs makes touching necessary, some people become more physically affectionate after Alzheimer's sets in.

One Sunday afternoon something unusual occurred: Sam offered to shave his father. At first, Mr. Kessler declined, but, sensing that his own hand was no longer steady, he hesitantly agreed. So Sam placed a stool in front of the bathroom sink and Mr. Kessler sat down. Sam then lathered his face and picked up a disposable razor. Watching them from the doorway, I noticed that once Mr. Kessler felt the warmth of Sam's fingers and the stroke of the razor, he began to enjoy himself. And Sam took pleasure in Mr. Kessler's unabashed delight at being pampered. "You're like a professional barber," Mr. Kessler said, chuckling as Sam finished up. "I should pay you." And then, when Sam wiped away the last of the lather, Mr. Kessler leaned into him and sighed, "Oh, that's good."

Although Mr. Kessler often forgot these moments, whenever Sam would say, "How about a nice shave?" he immediately put down his newspaper and joined Sam in the bathroom. Sam, I knew, looked forward to those fifteen minutes when he and his father could be together, and so it came as a jolt when during one of their sessions, Mr. Kessler, after telling Sam that he should be paid, casually added, "You need the money, don't you? Your hobby keeps you poor."

Taken aback, Sam felt a familiar surge of anger and quickly stepped away from the sink.

Mr. Kessler, unsure what had happened, turned his head and asked, "What's wrong? Why did you stop?"

Sam said nothing. Stolidly, he began shaving his father again.

Alzheimer's not only kept Mr. Kessler's image of himself intact, it also preserved an outdated image of Sam. Almost three decades had passed since Sam had been young and struggling, but Mr. Kessler now mostly lived in a past in which Sam's professional setbacks still tugged at him. At this stage of the disease, it was hard to know whether it was Alzheimer's or Mr. Kessler's selective memory that prompted his words. It's not uncommon, after all, for memory loss to collude with a person's preexisting and skewed sense of reality. Relating all this to me, Sam said something I would eventually hear from many caregivers: "He remembers what he wants to remember."

Over the years, I have encountered a lot of anger from caregivers. Sam was just one of many whose anger was constantly being rekindled by a patient's moving in and out of awareness. It's almost axiomatic that in troubled relationships, caregivers would rather hold on to their anger than accept the pain of losing someone when issues are still unresolved. And this reluctance to let go is only exacerbated by a disease that creates just enough ambiguity in a patient's behavior to keep caregivers from facing their grief.

One evening, as Sam helped his father get into bed, Mr. Kessler looked up and said in a kindly tone: "Who are you?"

Startled, Sam replied, "Your son."

"My son?" Mr. Kessler said wonderingly. "How long have you been my son?"

"Well, I guess sixty-two years now," Sam said, feeling both alarmed and amused.

Mr. Kessler's eyes widened. "Sixty-two years you've been my son and only *now* you're telling me?"

Sam laughed. "Well, sometimes it slips my mind."

Seeing his son laugh caused Mr. Kessler to laugh as well.

Later, a grim-looking Sam found me in the kitchen. "I'm a jerk," he muttered. "Why do I continue arguing with him? He doesn't even know who I am."

But he argued precisely because he didn't know what his father knew. A patient's memory of people and events, after all, does not just decamp when a degenerative disorder appears. Not only is memory stored in different places in the brain, there are also different kinds of memory. There is *explicit* memory that retains information: people, places, objects, and events. And there is *implicit* memory that safeguards skills, habits, expertise, music retention, preferences, and emotional associations. When amnesia patients in one experiment were given an electric shock while shaking hands, the following day they did not remember the person whose hand they shook (*explicit* memory), but they still hesitated when shaking that person's hand (*implicit* memory).

Dementia patients may likewise not remember a name

or a relationship, but the emotions (love, dislike, trust) associated with a person often remain. And what remains can be a saving grace but also a source of frustration. It's this implicit memory that allows them to speak and act in ways that are consistent with pre-dementia behaviors. For instance, patients who are also diabetic often sneak cookies and snacks right after a meal. They "sneak" because they sense it's wrong and they'll get in trouble if caught. And since "sneaking" implies awareness, caregivers might feel justified in scolding them even though they know they shouldn't.

Then again, shouldn't we make peace with the fact that patients remember some things but not others? But this is hard to do. Our mind abhors ambiguity, and as long as a patient's memory flickers on and off, we tend to see what we want to see. As I continued to observe Sam's seesawing reactions to his father's intermittent and fluctuating recall, I realized that it's not the absence of a memory system that frustrates and confounds caregivers but rather its fragmentation.

GIVEN ITS FANTASTICAL PREMISE, IT'S easy to forget that "Funes the Memorious" is not only about a singular young man from Uruguay; it is also about the man who spends an entire night with him. And because the narrator has a "normal" memory, he's unable at first to discern the chasm that exists between them. But soon it dawns on him that communication with Funes is nearly impossible. Funes's consummate memory makes him incapable of thinking as we understand it. His memories flow together so immaculately that he cannot differentiate past from present. He is actually disturbed by the fact "that a dog at three-fourteen (seen in profile) should have the same name as the dog at three-fifteen." It is also incomprehensible to him that the generic term *dog* "embraces so many unlike specimens of differing sizes and different forms."

We, thankfully, are not Funes: *Our* thoughts rely on concepts and categories in order to make sense of a world our memory cannot fully retain. But for Funes, whose memory is limitless, there is no cognitive incentive to convert the specific into the general. Memory, then, is not simply about remembering, and memory loss is not simply about forgetting. An altered memory is about more than pluses and minuses, deficits and surpluses. A dramatic change in memory changes everything because memory has a hand in everything. Memory is so integrated into every aspect of life—from thinking, to communicating, to forming and sustaining relationships, to creating continuity, meaning, and coherence—that its disappearance is incomprehensible. We simply have no cognitive framework that allows for its absence in others.

Human beings did not evolve to function in isolation, and in fact each person's cognition is dependent on the cognitive faculties of those around them. So when one person's memory is impaired, those close to him or her also become disoriented. Not only do we expect people's memories to work as ours do, we *need* to believe that memories are shared. Without this assumption, we couldn't form bonds of affection or trust or, conversely, feelings of antipathy or fear—all of which, in evolutionary terms, are necessary for survival. Because our expectation of memory is biological, we continue to rely on it even when we know it's gone.

For instance: Whenever Mr. Kessler broke his promise to stop fiddling with the light fixtures, Sam would be incredulous.

"You told me you wouldn't touch the wires or the outlets," he'd reprimand him. "You promised me!"

To which Mr. Kessler would typically reply, "What are you talking about? I never said that."

Having watched this scene play out repeatedly, I realized that no image of his father's shrunken hippocampus could alter Sam's expectations. In fact, most caregivers cannot refrain from shouting, "Don't you remember?"—a question that baffles practically everyone including the caregiver, who more than anyone else knows the patient cannot remember.

But to assume that caregivers can easily abandon the expectation of memory is also unfair. Given the way a "normal" memory functions, memory loss in someone we know well feels less like a neurological deficit than an act of betrayal. After all, when patients forget, it's the caregivers who end up feeling erased, their words, efforts, and sacrifices often going unacknowledged and even denied by their patients. It's why so many caregivers feel they're being gaslighted. Without the other person's memory working alongside our own, collaborating with us on facts and events, we're left shaky and unsure of what's real, of what's to be trusted and not trusted.

Memory doesn't even need to be grievously impaired for us to feel betrayed by a loved one's recollections. Aren't the worst fights often those begun by strikingly different memories of a shared experience? Because memory does not exist to serve "objective" reality but rather to create meaningful narratives, it makes sense that we can't count on other people's recollections to mirror our own. In healthy relationships, significant narratives are shared, making it easier to withstand the occasional, inevitable dissonance. But in relationships that are not healthy to begin with, the biases and capriciousness of memory can be used as weapons to dismiss and invalidate another person's reality and sense of self.

This is what makes Alzheimer's disease at once uncanny and maddeningly familiar. When people's memory disappears, their narratives become even more essential, filling in the blanks for the experiences that are being lost. And if these narratives contain rigid and belittling perceptions about a caregiver, they can make a relationship increasingly fraught. Memory loss does not just create ambiguity, it impedes the possibility of growth, of repair, of accountability, of achieving closure. For Sam and his father, two people who had always lived in different realities, Alzheimer's allowed them moments of unusual intimacy even as it widened the gap between them.

2

"The Weak Child"

Why It's So Hard to Change Our Responses

One morning a traveling salesman by the name of Gregor Samsa awakens from troubled dreams and discovers that he has turned into a "monstrous verminous bug." Oddly, he doesn't seem alarmed. He lies in bed and takes stock of his armor-plated belly and dozens of wriggling legs. He's a bug, but he seems more concerned that he can't turn onto his side. Suddenly he notices how late it is. He has a train to catch. He tries to get up, but his tiny legs and disproportionately large body make it difficult.

When Gregor finally emerges, the reactions of his family are both hysterical and banal. Everyone assumes the bug is Gregor but no one makes the slightest effort to question or comfort him. The days pass and Gregor grows accustomed to his new body. He eats spoiled food and learns to maneuver around the house. Willing as ever to accommodate his family, he makes himself invisible by squeezing into crevices. And because nothing much was ever expected of him, except a paycheck, his chirps and cries go unnoticed or misunderstood.

One day, Gregor overhears his sister pleading with their parents to get rid of him. She insists they stop treating him as their son. His parents seem sympathetic to her pleas, but this doesn't anger him. Instead, he's moved by her words. Hating the idea of being a burden, Gregor, in what seems like a final act of familial devotion, expires that very night. In the morning he's found covered in trash with bits of apple sticking to his shell.

IN A CREAKY OLD HOUSE in Jericho, Long Island, Mila Rivkin would regularly burst into her daughter and son-in-law's bedroom, looking for her stockings. "Find them!" she'd demand in a high-pitched voice. "My stockings are missing." When her daughter, Lara, didn't feel like crying from exhaustion, she'd laugh, because these particular stockings were hard to miss. Made from heavy Soviet wool, they seemed to weigh fifteen pounds. Mila was obsessed with them, as she was with most of her possessions. Her towels, for example: She had a different one for each part of her body, because some towels left places feeling either too damp or too dry. And heaven forbid you should ever hand her the wrong hairbrush, napkin, or teacup.

Lara had fantasies of burning her mother's things, but she kept her temper in check. Lara's husband, Misha, was not always so restrained. He regarded his mother-in-law as an attention-seeking, self-centered little girl, and sometimes when Mila showed up in the bedroom, he'd gleefully announce that he was wearing her stockings. Mila, never big on jokes, especially at her own expense, would angrily wave him off before launching into another fretful rant.

Mila's behavior was typical of someone with Alzheimer's. Her repetitive badgering, lack of emotional control, iffy memory, and self-absorption were obvious signs. And yet Mila did not have Alzheimer's at the time. She simply possessed those human flaws barely distinguishable from Alzheimer's symptoms. And, as is also true of most people, her annoying traits did not define her. She may have been demanding, self-involved, and needy, but she was also warm, generous, and incapable of holding a grudge.

It would be another six years, after Mila's husband developed Parkinson's, that actual symptoms of Alzheimer's appeared. But even then, Mila seemed unchanged. She continued to dote on her husband, unfazed by his mood swings, helping him to undress and tenderly kissing his neck as lovingly as ever.

When her husband passed away, however, Mila's symptoms escalated. Without someone to anchor her, she began to lean into some of her less appealing qualities, and gradually it became apparent that something was wrong. If it wasn't her stockings she wanted, it was a piece of bread, or a bowl of soup, or her hat, or the iron to press her favorite scarf. Because her memory was now spotty, the same demand came up every few minutes. Her voice, quavering with anxiety, had always distressed Lara, and now that her requests were incessant and delivered with a panting breathlessness, Mila sounded as if she were drowning, and Lara felt as if she were drowning alongside her.

Even when Mila wasn't accosting her daughter with questions, the house was rarely quiet. Alone in her room, Mila paced back and forth, with an irregular, limping gait typical of many Alzheimer's victims, and each shuffling step felt like an interrogation: Where is my hat? Where is my purse? Where are my keys? And should Lara awaken in the middle of the night, sleep was over. She'd lie in bed waiting to be summoned. Her only break came when she was at work or when Mila was at the adult care center.

But daycare also created problems. After a few weeks, Mila began to return home full of grievances about the staff and the other seniors. "They mock me," she'd say. "They talk behind my back. They torment me because they know I don't have any brains."

One night, after dinner, when Misha wasn't around, she whispered fearfully to Lara, "They're trying to control me with their thoughts. That's why I'm like this."

Her mother's helplessness and paranoia immediately disarmed Lara, washing away her anger and impatience. Gently, she assured Mila that she would take care of everything in the morning. In fact, she'd go to the senior center and talk to the people there.

"Tomorrow?" Mila responded with mocking bitterness. "Tomorrow I could be dead!"

And suddenly Lara was dealing not with a mind in distress, but with her mother's usual sense of entitlement, her expectation that Lara drop everything and come to her assistance.

"At this rate," Lara replied with uncharacteristic harshness, "I'm going to go first."

Mila gasped and tearfully shook her head. "Heaven forbid! Heaven forbid!" she cried. It took half the night to calm her down.

LARA CAME TO SEE ME about two months after Mila had been diagnosed. She was petite and pale, with intense, dark blue eyes. Sitting in an armchair across from me, she seemed coiled in place, as though it were painful to sit still. Even though she appeared to be fully engaged when we spoke, a part of her seemed to be elsewhere. It was only later I realized that Lara was always expecting to be interrupted. She was clearly not used to being the focus of attention, and when I asked her if she was comfortable, she gave me a small, hesitant smile suggesting that comfort was something long forgotten.

Lara was worried. Lately, she found herself reacting to Mila in ways she could neither explain nor condone. Although she continued to indulge her mother, she sometimes found herself giving in to perverse stirrings—muttering under her breath, making sarcastic remarks, pretending not to hear when Mila called—the kind of things that she had once chided her husband for.

Misha, on the other hand, no longer seemed put out by Mila's behavior. Once she had been diagnosed, he began to research the disease, and his feelings toward her changed. Now it was his wife's behavior that he found baffling. He'd remind her that Mila was sick and not to expect too much from her.

"So now he is the good guy," Lara said, looking bemused.

"Of course, he is," I said. "He's not the one your mother is obsessed with. He can afford to be charitable."

Lara laughed in agreement, but only for a moment. For the first time in her life, she was purely angry at her mother. Not only was this kind of anger alien to her, it troubled her that she could feel this way.

I asked her to give me other examples of what upset her. Somewhat bashfully, she confessed that Mila had taken to compulsively referring to herself as "the weak child," as in "Did you know I was the weak child of the family?" or "It's not my fault. I was always the weak child." Although Lara had heard variations of this line her entire life, she now found it unbearable. But what troubled her even more was her inability to suppress her irritation.

Why, I wanted to know, did she find this phrase so aggravating? Lara shrugged. She didn't know and didn't feel it was worth exploring. What mattered to her was her lack of patience. How could she get so worked up over a few innocent words? she asked me. I suspected the phrase was far from innocent.

MILA RIVKIN, I LEARNED, WAS born in Ukraine, in 1922, in the town of Berdychiv. She came from a close-knit family, but unlike her two sisters, she was small and sickly, so she was affectionately dubbed "the weak child." Walking home from school one day, she noticed a crowd of people. She stopped to ask what was going on, but no one would meet her gaze. Finally, someone came forward and told her that her father had been run over by a car. But this made no sense. The town had only two cars and she had never seen either one of them. How could such a thing happen?

When Mila arrived home, she sensed immediately from her mother's somber expression that it was true and that everything was about to change. At twelve, she had to drop out of school in order to work and look after her mother. And though she was a kindly, good-natured child, she resented her new obligations. Instead of being tended to, she now had to tend to someone else. She had lost what the British psychologist John Bowlby calls a "secure base," someone who represents a safe haven during times of stress.

As it happens, human beings and other mammals are born with an innate attachment system that motivates them to seek proximity. This adaptive behavioral function helps alleviate stress and ensures survival by "notifying" attachment figures to be present and responsive. Children who are deprived of a secure base, or who have parents who do not function as one, tend to develop defensive coping strategies. Some become "avoidantly attached"—that is, rigidly self-reliant and distrustful of close relationships. Others, like Mila, become "anxiously attached," terrified of being abandoned again. Such children become overly dependent on others and tend to react to small stressors as though they were catastrophes.

These coping mechanisms or attachment styles can extend well beyond childhood and affect how we move through the world. They influence our personality development, our attitude toward ourselves and others, and of course the relationships we form with our own children.

When Mila grew up, she immediately set about having a family. She wanted a child not because she wanted someone to nurture, but because she wanted to *be* nurtured. And so, unlike most "securely attached" parents, who act as a secure base for their children, Mila turned her daughter into the secure base that she had been deprived of. For Mila, the world was a chaotic, scary place, and Lara was her lifeline. As Lara told me during one of our first meetings, she had often accompanied her mother on late-night shopping trips because Mila felt safer with her small daughter at her side.

Because it was all she had ever known, Lara simply took for granted her mother's neediness and fearful exclamations of "What will people think?" or "What is to become of me?" From a very young age she had learned how to ease her mother's anxieties by assuring her that she wasn't alone, that she, Lara, was there to help. Even after she attended university in Moscow, got married, and emigrated to America, she never felt free of her mother's anxieties. Mila's singular uneasiness remained in her thoughts, but what could Lara do about it, living on another continent?

It was a constant worry, the depth of which she did not truly understand—until one day, ten years after leaving Russia, she opened a letter from the Department of State that granted permission for her parents to come to America. She burst into tears, relieved by the thought that they would soon be together again. No longer would she be depriving her mother of a lifeline.

But when Mila was diagnosed with Alzheimer's, Lara felt thwarted. Mila, it seemed, had officially been given license to be infantile. Lara knew, of course, that Mila couldn't help herself, that her memory, attention span, and self-control were all impaired, yet somehow it was hard to believe and even harder to stomach. Her mother had Alzheimer's, but had a metamorphosis really occurred?

WHEN I FIRST READ "The Metamorphosis," some twenty years ago, I felt a natural dislike toward a family too self-involved to deal with a stricken son. Transformed into an insect, Gregor scuttles on the ground and communicates only by emitting small cries. Yet the family's response is comically underwhelming. After the initial shock wears off, the parents and sister fall back on their usual passivity, self-pity, and sense of entitlement.

Naturally, I assumed it was their farcical self-involvement that hardened them to Gregor's transformation. But having met many caregivers like Lara, whose life is defined by sacrifice and solicitude, I've come to see that Kafka's family portrait is emblematic of many families—that is to say, the more unsettling the disruption, the more they revert to entrenched patterns of behavior. Kafka merely took a preexisting family dynamic to its absurd conclusion.

Alzheimer's victims may not mutate into insects, but they do change. Nonetheless, in case after case, patient and caregiver often continue to interact as they always have. Most caregivers, of course, have more self-awareness than the Samsas, but this doesn't stop them from regressing into habitual familial roles. Such patterns continue because they are at the mercy of something deceptively powerful: the unconscious.

Although today a byword in psychological/philosophical circles, the unconscious was not always esteemed. Greeted at first with astonishment, an unknown country to be explored and mined for treasure, it attracted a great many educated people who decided that psychoanalysis would help them discover their inner selves. Freud's psychoanalytic netherworld was both scary and appealing; it not only seemed to explain why we have specific urges, it also explored why those urges worked at cross-purposes with civilization. In order for society to function, a certain part of the unconscious had to be repressed and/or sublimated.

But then, around the middle of the twentieth century, a sea change occurred. A new wave of psychologists began to apply a hard-nosed empirical approach to the study of unconscious mental processes, thus ushering in the "cognitive revolution." People still dutifully reclined on a psychoanalyst's couch, but in academic circles it was generally agreed that many mental processes occur without our knowledge, guiding much of what we think and do. Freud's assertion that consciousness is only "the tip of the iceberg" proved to be truer than anyone had anticipated, though perhaps not in the way he intended. This new, more quotidian unconscious emphasized the cognitive and perceptual day-to-day operations that hummed along independently of consciousness.

Moreover, these unconscious processes, as Timothy Wilson writes in *Strangers to Ourselves,* are "part of the architecture of the brain," influencing judgment, feelings, language, perception, and decision-making, the better to make us function more efficiently. This "adaptive unconscious," a term first coined by the social psychologist Daniel M. Wegner, allows us to quickly size up our environment and respond without interference from consciousness, which works more slowly and requires more mental energy. And because the adaptive unconscious works below the radar, we tend to give consciousness credit for most of our thoughts and actions.

One might picture consciousness obliviously working alongside invisible zombies who quietly perform what the conscious mind believes it's doing. Indeed, unconscious processes are sometimes referred to as "zombie subsystems," automated drudges that take over when we perform such routine tasks as combing our hair, washing the dishes, turning off the lights—tasks that don't require much awareness.

Yet many of these unconscious processes can also involve sophisticated thinking and behavior, especially when they align with a particular skill or area of expertise. Thus, people—even those with intellectually complex or mechanically precise jobs—can continue performing at a high level during the early and even middle stages of dementia disorders. This, naturally, can obscure the extent of their cognitive impairment from themselves, while creating unreasonable expectations in everyone around them.

Therapists, lawyers, plumbers, and academics may look and sound as though their mental cylinders are pegging away, but it's unconscious processes that are actually doing most of the work. It's no wonder that caregivers are deceived—we generally believe that judgment, thinking, and character are all guided by conscious and deliberate "higher" processes, and so we're puzzled when dementia patients do not seem particularly diminished.

WHEN MILA RIVKIN DEVELOPED ALZHEIMER'S, the disease did not immediately change how her family saw her. Crucial aspects of personality that derive from unconscious processes—temperament, preferences, characteristic responses, sociability—stayed more or less the same. To Lara and Misha, Mila still "felt" like Mila. Her tiresome expressions and dubious narratives did not cease; they only redoubled, to help her cope. As was true of Mr. Kessler, when Mila's complex cognition began to disappear, she clung even more tightly to the unconscious scripts that she'd always relied on and that had always defined her.

So when Mila repeated one of her patented lines about being "the weak child," Lara saw only her mother, not a disease. And when Lara delivered a taunt or a rebuke, it was directed at her mother, not at the disease. Mila, unaware, of course, that she was assailing Lara with incessant remarks and questions, only looked blank.

MILA: Where do you think you're going?
LARA: Where do I ever go? To the store.
MILA: To the store, to the store. And what am I supposed to do? Who is going to take care of me while you're gone? I am alone all day.

LARA: What are you talking about? We spent the whole day together. I walked with you, gave you a bath, we had dinner.

MILA: So I am a burden?

LARA: Mom, what do you want from me?

MILA: Have I eaten? I would like a piece of bread.

LARA: I've already told you—that's why I have to go to the store. We're out of the bread you like.

MILA: You're going to the store? And what's going to happen to me?

LARA: You'll stay home.

MILA: Alone, like a dog.

(*Seeing her daughter leaving, she became more agitated.*)

MILA: Where are you going?

LARA: For the hundredth time, I'm going to the store!

MILA: And what am I going to do?

Naturally, Lara was frustrated. Like so many other caregivers, she began to mimic the very symptoms that oppressed her. For one thing, she found that she was repeating herself. Ironically, such "contagion" may be due in part to the brain's plasticity. The healthy brain is miraculously, wonderfully adaptable. But instead of allowing caregivers to change their habits and expectations to cope with dementia disorders, it can make them as stubborn and prone to repetition as their patients. In *The Brain That Changes Itself,* the psychiatrist Norman Doidge makes use of the sledding analogy devised by the neurologist Alvaro Pascual-Leone to explain why rigidity occurs. Imagine you're on a sled atop a hill of fresh snow. You sled down the hill, climb back up, and then either take the same path or forge a new one. The options are infinite, but each time you take the same route, the tracks made by the sled deepen and harden, and the more well-defined they become, the easier it is to ride down that particular path again. Repetition thus begets more repetition.

In cases of dementia disorder, repetition is an obvious symptom, but what ensnares caregivers is that such repetition is not just the product of pathology. The patient's fixations, demands, pet phrases, needling remarks, and constant phone calls are natural attachment behaviors that emerge in response to stress. Alzheimer's especially can create an internal climate so overrun by confusion, anxiety, and unidentifiable loss that the attachment system becomes overloaded, driving victims to seek a secure base, searching obsessively for an absent parent, home, doll, article of clothing—anything that represents security.

Lara had been Mila's secure base long before Mila fell victim to a disease. Alzheimer's didn't suddenly change this; on the contrary, the disease only heightened Mila's anxious attachment style. The same holds true for patients with an avoidant attachment style. Instead of seeking closeness, they can become more mistrustful, less willing to accept help, and increasingly insistent on maintaining their independence. In effect, the behaviors that caregivers see day to day are those they've witnessed their whole lives—only now they seem more pronounced.

When Mila called for Lara every five minutes, it wasn't only because she forgot they had just spoken; it was also because her attachment system made her desperate for comfort. And when she repeatedly referred to herself as "the weak child," it wasn't only because she'd forgotten what she just said; it was also because her coping mechanism led her to emphasize her vulnerability and helplessness, the better to appeal to an attachment figure. Even when she was well, Mila had demanded attention and closeness. But now, in thrall to the disease, when her whole world was a dark, empty street, she held on even more tightly to Lara. And Lara once again became the little girl whose job it was to make her mother feel safe in the darkness.

The more Lara talked about her past, the more she relaxed. After several meetings, she settled back in her chair, finally looking as if she had nowhere else to go. One afternoon, she fell silent, and I did too, gratified that she was giving herself a moment to reflect, a moment entirely her own. When she spoke up, it was to tell me why the phrase "the weak child" felt so stifling. The constant refrain, she mused, not only served to infantilize Mila, it also strangely felt like an admonishment or a warning, as though to say: "Don't you forget what I have been through and don't you abandon me." So every time Lara acted unkind or impatient, she felt she was not just a bad daughter but also a "bad mom."

A good mother, Lara said with a touch of irony, would show more patience when Mila returned from daycare complaining about being ridiculed and rejected by the people at the center. Every afternoon when she came home, it was the same lament: "You should see how they treat me. Thank God you're here. Thank God. I don't know how I made it."

Hearing this, Lara's heart fell. She imagined Mila standing by herself at the adult care center, feeling disoriented and scared.

"You should see how they talk to me. No one is there to look after me. No one is there. No one cares."

But after a few loops of this, Lara would snap, "How can you say no one cares? All I do is make sure that every minute you're not alone."

Once the floodgates opened, Lara could not stop. Why didn't Mila recognize how much she did for her? Why didn't Mila understand that someone was there for her, had always been there for her? Why couldn't Mila appreciate the trouble she caused?

Mila, feeling attacked by her own daughter, could barely hold back her tears.

"Why are you shouting at me? Is it my fault I am still alive?"

Every morning Lara promised herself that she would let her mother bewail her misfortunes while she, the dutiful daughter, would calmly listen. But as soon as her mother started up, Lara, as if under a spell, retaliated, falling back on the same lines that she had fed her mother the day before and the day before that. Knowing that her response was pointless and feeling ridiculous did not prevent the same words from pouring out of her.

Lara is hardly alone in this response pattern. When a patient's attachment system is constantly clamoring to be soothed, a caregiver's own attachment system can't help but get triggered. Because she had grown up with such a clinging mother, Lara's emotional equilibrium was directly tied to her mother's. In soothing her mother, she soothed herself.

Once Alzheimer's entered the picture, Mila's anxieties became an alarm that could not be shut off. And since there was never a reprieve from her mother's distress, there could be no escape from her own.

In effect, Lara's own attachment system also became overloaded, and she, too, reverted to her own typical coping pattern—reflexively trying to fix her mother. Alzheimer's had created a bottomless well of need in Mila, making Lara feel that nothing she did was ever enough. The disease only amplified the volume of what Lara had been hearing most of her life: her mother's insatiable demands. But it was only now that she began to chafe against them.

THE OBSTACLES TO CHANGING A patient's behavior are clear, but those facing caregivers are less evident. In order for caregivers to resist old habits when reacting to their patients' demands, they need to switch over from unconscious to conscious responses. Sounds simple, but the brain makes it difficult. The brain's objective, after all, is not to be wise or right or even reasonable, but to conserve energy. Why spend energy on pricey conscious activities when "cheaper" unconscious processes are handy? Under duress, our brains become especially frugal and we fall back on old patterns of behavior, and the more we resort to these patterns, the deeper our neural grooves become and the harder it is to choose a different path.

Just as Gregor's family responded to his bizarre incarnation in their characteristically selfish, unfeeling ways, caregivers settle into their own familiar grooves with patients. And in intimate, entangled relationships, our neural paths converge with those of our patients'; their repetitive behaviors beget our own. How could it be otherwise? Lara's attachment system had been shaped by the very person she was now caring for. So Alzheimer's acts like a serpent's tail, flicking one person's emotional responses back at the other.

Growing up in the former Soviet Union, in a cramped apartment, sleeping three to a room, Lara had longed for solitude before she even knew what it meant. Today she lives in a house of her own—but Mila lives with her, and though she has her own room, her plaintive voice roams through the house. "What's to become of me?" "What will people think of me?" "What am I to do?"—questions that have always triggered Lara's claustrophobia. But it was only after the disease entered the house that the repetition began to taunt her, an oppressive reminder that she was stuck in the role she had occupied ever since she could walk.

3

Dementia Blindness

Why It Takes So Long
to See the Disease

THERE IS A DECEPTIVELY SIMPLE OPTICAL ILLUSION THAT consistently fools us. The Müller-Lyer illusion consists of two parallel lines, one with fins pointing inward and the other with fins extending outward. The lines are of equal length,

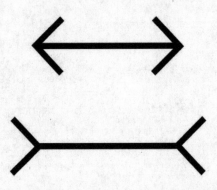

yet no matter how many times we measure them, the one with the fins diverging will always appear longer. This tension between what we know conceptually and what we perceive instinctively is built into us and is, I believe, at the heart of the caregiver's dilemma.

Caregivers may realize their parents or spouses suffer from dementia, but in many cases it does not inhibit them from reacting emotionally and erratically to their patient's misconduct or delusions. Knowing better does not necessarily make caregivers behave better. I encountered this phenomenon so often (even with well-informed caregivers) that I began to wonder if there wasn't a neurological component to a family member's inability to accept the full implications of cognitive impairment.

In *Thinking, Fast and Slow,* the psychologist Daniel Kahneman explains what's at work here. He postulates two modes of thinking. System 1 is our automatic mode of thinking; it runs effortlessly, forms immediate impressions, and produces visceral and emotional reactions. This unconscious process, which Kahneman dubs "fast thinking," is almost impossible to suppress. System 1 recruits our intuitions, biases, and assumptions and makes us susceptible to various visual and cognitive pitfalls, such as the Müller-Lyer illusion.

System 2 is our more deliberate mode of thinking; it works at a conceptual remove and is slower to pronounce judgment. We can think of System 1 as the loud-mouthed uncle who knows the answer to everything and System 2 as the egghead professor given to murmuring, "I'm afraid I don't know about that," or "Maybe we should think things over." And perhaps if System 2 had more sway over us, it would help us see what we *know* to be true. Although dementia does not play with lines and angles, it does something even trickier to disguise itself.

On a fall day a few years ago, an experienced social worker came to see me. Jasmine Hines was thirty-six, a tall, pretty, willowy woman with large hazel eyes that often seemed on the verge of welling up. Soft-spoken and even-keeled, she was unflinching when assessing her strengths and weaknesses. She was also honest with others, which helped when dealing with at-risk kids. But after her father, Stewart, died of cancer, she quit her job to take care of her mother, Pat.

When Jasmine spoke about Stewart, her voice brightened with affection and flashes of humor. But when Pat's name came up, her voice became weary, almost deflated. She often thought about Stewart not just because she missed him, but because she had come to realize how much she had relied on him and how expertly he had hidden Pat's dementia from her. Even seeing her parents every day, Jasmine never suspected the extent of her mother's decline.

Now, looking back, she could identify both subtle and not-so-subtle clues. The time, for instance, that Pat got behind the wheel of her car and turned to Jasmine, saying, "I don't know what to do here." To which Jasmine had replied, "Okay, Mom, very funny." But when Pat opened the glove compartment, a list of instructions on how to start the car fell out. The note was in Stewart's handwriting.

Jasmine paused, as if to consider what she'd just told me. "That should have tipped me off, huh? Instead I just thought, 'How convenient. Daddy to the rescue.'"

"Did your father always come to the rescue?" I asked.

"Yes, he did. I should have seen what was happening. But I didn't want to deal with it, so I ignored it."

It pained me to see her blaming herself for something that most caregivers also miss. Although clear-cut signs of Alzheimer's—incoherence, sexual inappropriateness, getting lost in familiar places, paranoid delusions, even physical violence—are often present, family members still hesitate to make the leap to a neurological diagnosis. Patients, of course, don't need help in denying the disease. How can they keep track of symptoms when they can't remember things from moment to moment? For so many of them the disease creates and then hides behind cognitive impairment. But what about caregivers? Might not their denial have a neurological component? I believe this to be the case and have come to think of it as "dementia blindness."

By thinking about it in these terms, I was reminded of the real blind spot that exists in the human eye, at the point where the optic nerve exits the retina. At this one point in each eye there are no photoreceptors. In effect, there is a gap where sensory data is not registered. Nonetheless, when we look out into the world we perceive a complete picture. This is because the brain, using visual information at the borders of the blind spot, fills in the gap with what it *expects* to see. In a similar way, the brain conceals from us what it doesn't know with what it does know. It finds our preexisting emotional blind spot and exploits it.

As I listened to Jasmine, I began to grasp what her blind spot might be. When Stewart was on his deathbed, he had called Pat from the hospital and asked her to bring him a book. Jasmine, who was standing near her mother, saw that

Pat was becoming agitated during the call. She didn't know where the book was, Pat told Stewart. She didn't know if she could bring it to him. Jasmine was then startled to hear her father yelling over the phone that she had better find the book, and even more startled when Pat became outraged and began to yell back.

Dumbfounded, Jasmine pleaded, "Mom, Dad is dying. He's allowed to yell at you. When you're dying, you can do that."

Hesitantly, I asked Jasmine if she didn't think that Pat was already suffering from dementia.

She shrugged. "Hey, it was just Mom being Mom."

Maybe it was just Pat being Pat, but her confusion and anger were also classic signs of dementia. Although it troubled Jasmine that Pat had yelled at Stewart, it didn't occur to her to consider that her mother's confusion and anger might signal a neurological problem.

Once again I saw how hard it is to attribute a neurological cause to the speech and behaviors that have always colored our impressions of people. Caregivers are not just hampered by a patient's adaptive unconscious, which makes them seem less ill than they are; caregivers' own minds often misinterpret what's right in front of them. Patients may unknowingly help create the illusion that they're still okay, but it is the healthy mind that falls for the illusion. This susceptibility, which often goes unremarked, is fairly common; it might even be likened to the way we're fooled by an actual optical illusion.

Consider, for instance, the Hollow-Face illusion (see illustration on page 45). We see a convex face even though

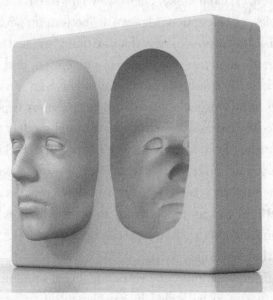

the lines of the face are actually concave. The face *looks* convex because our minds have plenty of experience with real faces, which are in fact convex. And this in turn leads to a *neural expectation* of convexity that is so strong that it trumps the sensory signal (i.e., concavity) itself.

So why does the eye see what the mind knows is wrong? According to the cognitive scientist Andy Clark, these visual mistakes are not glitches in the brain or even random errors. They are, in fact, neural tendencies that reveal something "right" about the brain even if it happens to be, in specific instances, mistaken about what is being viewed.

Traditionally, the perceptual system was believed to be passive or stimulus-driven, a view that reflects our intuitions about reality. We intuitively feel that we have direct access to the outside world and that all we need to do is sit back and let our senses, cameralike, click away. This passive, stimulus-driven view of perception is known as "bottom-up perception."

Today, however, we know that the brain isn't just along for the ride; it's an active participant in perception, and the visible world is the result of a compromise between sensory data and the mind's expectations based on previous experience. Because we naturally construct an internal model of reality, what we already know influences what is still to be known, if not always accurately. This tendency toward expectation-based perception is referred to as "top-down processing," and it sometimes causes expectations to override incoming sensory signals. A picture of a face can be concave, but it won't appear that way to us.

If our expectations can override reality, it's practically axiomatic that we'll be fooled by misperceptions more important than an optical illusion. Imagine being in the woods and coming across a bear. If we had no internal model of what woods or bears look like, we'd likely be dead by the time our mind could make sense of the data. Then again, we could be wrong. Perhaps the bear is actually an unusually large, bearish-looking dog. Nonetheless, we'd still think *Bear!* and run away, or perhaps play dead. Later we might feel embarrassed for overreacting, but it's a small price to pay. After all, our biological imperative is to survive, not to keep our pride intact or to prevent us from making inconsequential mistakes.

Preconceptions guide us subtly and persuasively. Without an internal model of the world, life would be too noisy, too ambiguous, too chaotic. With nothing to orient us, we'd get lost in endless details, or become confused by too much stimuli, or end up paralyzed by a surfeit of choices. Without experientially shaped expectations, we'd have to start from scratch with *every* interaction or impression. It would take us too long to figure out what was harmful or benign, who's a friend or a foe.

So just as memory is not built for accuracy, neither is perception, and the occasional error is surely worth our overall ability to function efficiently. Dementia blindness exists because we do more than merely observe the world around us. We interpret it, as Andy Clark notes, against "a rich background of prior knowledge." And it's precisely because we know our spouse or parent so well that dementia tricks us, making us see enough familiar cues to think that everything is fine.

The research of Nassim Nicholas Taleb seems to support this explanation. Taleb argues that we have a propensity to overlook the anomalous by creating "narrative fallacies" that impose coherence by tailoring unexpected phenomena to fit into our preexisting assumptions. In the same way that we make sense of the visual world (which sometimes means being fooled by it), we form expectations of the people around us, projecting narratives onto family members which obscure the evidence of their impairment. We unconsciously smooth out the anomalies dementia presents so that what looks like atypical behavior to an outsider feels like just another familiar assault to a caregiver. And just as we subconsciously impose preconceived expectations on the visual world, causing us to fall for optical illusions, we bend dementia symptoms to fit what we already know about our spouse or parent.

———

AFTER STEWART DIED, JASMINE MOVED into her parents' brownstone on Convent Avenue in Harlem. It's a large four-story building that feels somehow less imposing because of all the notes Scotch-taped to doors and walls: "DON'T LEAVE THE HOUSE WITHOUT TELLING SOMEONE." "DON'T YELL AT THE AIDES. THEY ARE HERE TO HELP." Over the years, I've seen similar notes in so many homes that I sometimes imagine them in every language all over the world, a universal attempt to create order out of chaos. Despite not being very effective, these domestic commandments are evidence of a battle of wills between patient and caregiver, each one fighting for a semblance of control.

In Jasmine's home, the kitchen had the most instructions: "DON'T TAKE FOOD OUT OF THE FREEZER." "LOOK AT THE MENU ON THE TABLE." "DON'T EAT JASMINE'S FOOD." The first time I visited Jasmine, she caught me studying the notes and I felt slightly embarrassed, as though I'd been caught eavesdropping.

As with many familial caregivers, there was a long and troubled history between child and parent. Pat's mother had worked too hard as a cleaning woman to pay her much attention, and her brothers considered her just a girl, unfit for the important things in life. As a result, Pat had always felt that she was on her own. She had worked long hours, earning a Ph.D. from an Ivy League school and becoming the only African American woman on the engineering faculty of a large university. And perhaps because she never received enough attention from her mother, Pat's love for her own kids took the form of pushing them—especially Jasmine, her only daughter—to succeed. They learned how to speak well, dress well, and do well. A-minuses in school were not good enough. They had to earn A's and A-pluses to win her approval.

When Jasmine alluded to her mother's impossible standards, she defended and bemoaned them in equal measure. Her mother had accomplished so much—why should she expect less from her children? But not all of Pat's parental methods were easy to justify. For example, when Jasmine was seven years old, Pat had put her on a diet of three glasses of milk and eight saltine crackers a day. Days one and two had passed without incident, but on the third day, while trying on dresses at Barney's, Jasmine fainted.

Seeing my horrified face at this point in the story, Jasmine said, half in earnest, "In fairness to my mom, she was on a diet with me."

Not surprisingly, Jasmine later developed an eating disorder. If she could stay thin, that was one thing she could do right. But her mother never once acknowledged that Jasmine had a problem. Did Pat know and purposely ignore it, or was an eating disorder not part of her generation's cultural vocabulary?

Jasmine's father, however, knew what was going on and gave Pat a book called *Mothers and Daughters with Eating Disorders*. Pat never glanced at it. She didn't refuse to look at it; she simply pretended it didn't exist.

"Do you think if she had read it, things would be different?" I asked.

"Well, maybe I wouldn't have called her a bitch yesterday."

"What happened?" I asked.

"Well," Jasmine said dryly, "she was acting like a bitch."

The flippant reply, of course, belied how terrible she felt about fighting with her mother. The fight, as I learned, was typical and centered on food. It began with Pat rummaging in the freezer. Finding her mother in front of the open refrigerator, Jasmine tried to close the door but was angrily shoved aside, hitting her head hard against the edge of the fridge. Pat didn't even notice.

JASMINE: Mom! Put the fish back in the freezer, please.

PAT: I want to see what we're having for dinner tomorrow.

JASMINE: Just look at the menu. What's the point of my making a menu if you don't look at it?

PAT: Who asked you to do that?

JASMINE: You did.

PAT: I *never* asked for it.

JASMINE: Yeah, Mommy, you did. And I do it for you, so please do this for me.

PAT: It's none of your business what I do with *my* freezer.

JASMINE: It's *our* freezer. Just put the fish back. We're going to have shrimp tomorrow.

PAT: How do you know?

JASMINE: Because I'm going to make it. Look at the menu.

(*Pat shrugged and continued rummaging in the freezer.*)

JASMINE: Mommy, put it back! If you take food out, it'll spoil.

PAT: You gonna tell me how to cook things? I've been cooking before you were born.

(*Pat removed a bag of chicken breasts and looked delighted.*)
JASMINE: Mommy, put that back. What do you need them for?
PAT: I want it out. I am the mama and you are the child! Why do you always have to make things so difficult?

Jasmine's head was throbbing, but it was Pat's final accusation that stung. She understood that Pat's confusion and rummaging were by-products of the disease, but part of her also believed that if Pat really cared about her, she would allow her at least one place in the house where she could exercise some control. But Pat didn't do that.

Jasmine ended the argument by walking away and then giving her mother the silent treatment.

Pat, of course, quickly forgot the entire episode and couldn't understand why Jasmine wasn't speaking to her. Shaken by her mother's hostile shove and her hurtful comment, Jasmine put up another sign: "VIOLENCE IS NOT THE ANSWER."

Telling me this, Jasmine went from being wryly amused to being deeply regretful. "God, I hate the guilt," she said slowly. "I hate it, I hate it."

THE THIRD TIME I MET with Jasmine, she asked me out of the blue if dementia makes people more selfish. I told her that dementia often makes people *appear* selfish, but that the root of their self-involvement lies in their inability to keep track of other people's needs and feelings. Even as I said this, I cringed at my clinical tone. My answer, like many answers that are technically correct, missed the point of the question. Luckily, Jasmine herself got straight to it: "It feels the same."

And it does. The problem for caregivers is that when patients appear the same, it is very hard not to treat them the same. So when spouses or parents act out, caregivers respond as though they're still healthy. In fact, many devise strategies to change their behavior. Jasmine's taped-up notes, Sam Kessler's insistence that his father repeat instructions three times: Both are typical methods to get patients to remember. "It works!" Sam assured me. "If he repeats things, it works."

"All the time?" I asked.

"Not every time," he conceded.

When I asked Jasmine if she thought her notes were effective, she was dubious. She knew that Alzheimer's affects attention span, but she wasn't ready to give up. "Sometimes the notes work," she said.

Initially, this supposition might seem baffling. Why rely on a strategy that yields inconsistent results? In a famous experiment, B. F. Skinner placed hungry pigeons in a box and gave them food at random. He observed that whatever the pigeons were doing before they were given food—cooing, hopping, bowing their heads, twirling in place—they would obsessively repeat in an attempt to trigger another reward. Skinner deduced that animals are prone to seeing cause and effect even when events are unrelated, and he went on to identify this inclination as the source of superstition, magical thinking, and ritualistic behavior.

He also found that when he gave rewards to mice at random, it made them more desperate to receive them than if the treats were administered consistently. Indeed, it became more difficult for them to unlearn what they were doing once the rewards stopped coming. The same might be said of human beings. Randomness creates a cognitive itch that needs to be scratched. People who run casinos and create gaming apps know that doling out rewards in unpredictable ways is what keeps users hooked.

What do Skinner's superstitious pigeons, obsessive mice, and addictive gaming apps have to do with caregiving? In a way, they mirror how we respond to patients who *sometimes* take their medicine, *sometimes* stick to a schedule, *sometimes* keep their promises, and *sometimes* keep their hands off food in accordance with our instructions. Our normal, selective memory fastens on those occasions when a strategy works, thereby creating a causal connection that isn't really there.

Why is unpredictability so unsettling? Why do we need to deny randomness? As the science writer Michael Shermer explains in *The Believing Brain,* we look for patterns because making associations and seeing connections improves our chances of survival. It's safer, after all, to believe that an unfamiliar sight, sound, smell, or shadow is linked to danger as opposed to finding it random or harmless. And since it's far better to be wrong than unsafe, we sometimes make false, even bizarre connections.

Imposing order on random events is such a powerful instinct that psychologists have found that when people experience a loss of control, they're more likely to see patterns where none exist. Alzheimer's takes that control away not just from the patients but also from caregivers. In the early and middle stages of the disease, the patient might have fluctuating moods, variable cognitive capacity, and erratic memory, all of which create a chaotic environment. So even when they expect these behavioral changes, caregivers will weave narratives to explain them away. After all, the mind naturally bends what is unpredictable into what feels familiar. In this way, Alzheimer's hides behind the unpredictability it creates.

Jasmine summed it up perfectly: "She's tricky, my mother. She has Alzheimer's when it's convenient and doesn't when it's not." For Jasmine, Pat's occasional inability to follow directions did not feel like the random workings of a sick brain; it was in keeping with Pat's tendency to do what she wanted to do while discounting Jasmine's needs.

Once again: Awareness of the disease does not prevent it from hiding in plain sight. As Kahneman explains, cognitive illusions can be just as convincing as visual ones; and cognitive illusions associated with dementia are, I believe, particularly seductive—because while optical illusions go away or don't matter when we don't look at them, dementia disorders bring us *into* the picture, since these illusions are perpetuated by *both* patient and caregiver. Patients, in fact, invite misperceptions, because before Alzheimer's erodes aspects of who they are, it can, as we have seen, magnify who they have always been.

When Pat's Alzheimer's became a daily fact of life, Jasmine channeled the A-student mentality her mother had instilled in her. She attended seminars, read the right books, and made the necessary accommodations to cope with the disease. All this came at a cost to her social life, job, and independence. So when Pat accused Jasmine of always making things difficult, it not only hurt, it also suggested that she had not done enough.

Even though it was Alzheimer's that prevented Pat from logically following her daughter's arguments or absorbing her instructions, her resistance didn't feel as if it was *just* neurological. Although Pat could not cognitively follow Jasmine's instructions, her reactions conformed to her old coping style: When things are difficult, *never* accept blame. The most painful instance of this for Jasmine was her mother's refusal to acknowledge Jasmine's eating disorder. If she didn't acknowledge it, she didn't have to understand her own role in her daughter's illness. And perhaps this is why Jasmine, who has always been sensible and forgiving, was unable to accept Pat's high-handedness in the kitchen.

These squabbles over food might seem superficial, but Jasmine felt them as a deep injustice. Pat, after all, had played a significant role in Jasmine's need to control her food intake, and here was Pat taking that control away. Although Pat had never acknowledged Jasmine's illness, Jasmine's life was now being ruled by her mother's affliction. No wonder the disease became invisible to Jasmine during their arguments. Invariably, a caregiver's most susceptible blind spot is an old familial wound.*

---

* As occurs in many families, a patient's need to control declines as the disease progresses, which naturally leads to a lessening of tensions. Like others who graciously consented to speak to me, Jasmine shared a time that was most fraught with conflicts and recriminations. In time, however, a more loving and gentle dynamic emerged between Jasmine and her mom.

4

Chekhov and the Left-Brain Interpreter

Why We Believe That the Person We Used to Know Is Still There

IN GREENWICH VILLAGE, ALONG ONE OF THE PLEASANT STREETS that converge near the Jefferson Market Garden, there is a small Italian restaurant. It's the sort of restaurant that used to be more fashionable in the Village: intimate, dimly lit, with red-and-white-checked tablecloths and candles in Chianti bottles. Sometimes, after work, Elizabeth Horn would meet her husband, Mitch, for a cocktail and dinner. Elizabeth would usually arrive to find Mitch highball in hand and joking with a waiter. They'd kiss and she'd order a Tanqueray and tonic. They had been friends before becoming romantically involved and bantered back and forth without missing a beat. Anyone looking at their table might well have envied them, never suspecting that Elizabeth dreaded these pleas-ant get-togethers and their aftermath.

Elizabeth, a tall, elegant woman in her late fifties, talks about those evenings in a composed, confiding tone, which only makes her story more uncanny. Because once the meal was over, Mitch would invariably give her a wary, skeptical look and say, "Now you'll go to your place and I'll go to mine." Hearing these words, Elizabeth would nod meekly, duck into the bathroom, take off her heels, put on a pair of sneak-ers, and run out. She'd cross the street, wait for Mitch to emerge—making sure he was headed in the right direction—and then hurry home to wait for him.

It always struck her how normal Mitch appeared, casu-ally strolling along in his sport jacket and Rolling Stones T-shirt, looking pretty much like the man she had fallen in love with. It was herself she barely recognized: the nervous, frazzled woman hiding behind lampposts, following a man who looked so at ease in the world. Then, with a burst of speed, she managed to get back to their apartment a few minutes before he did.

Arriving home, Mitch always gave her the same cheerful greeting: "Hey, honey, how are you?" He had already forgot-ten their rendezvous.

"This is something out of *The Twilight Zone*," I said the first time I heard the story.

Elizabeth sighed. "It gets worse, believe me. It was hor-rendous, surreal, and I knew I had to do it all over again the next day. Every day I dreaded the night and every night was a nightmare."

The nightmare would officially begin after Mitch had

made himself comfortable. Without any warning, he'd look up from a magazine or the TV, stare at Elizabeth, and ask her to leave. Calmly at first, he'd order her out of her own home. When she tried to convince him that she *was* home, he'd scoff. How could it be her home, when *he* lived there? Although he sensed that they knew each other, he had forgotten they were married. Moreover, he felt threatened by her presence.

When Mitch first began to act this way, Elizabeth had done her best to plead her case. She'd point to things in the apartment and remind him of where they came from. "Look," she'd say. "Our wedding picture, see?"

Unfazed, Mitch would reply, "Yeah? You must have planted it there."

"What about these?" she'd say, waving forms and letters addressed to both of them.

"Well, maybe we were married once, but not now. Sorry, but you have to go."

Adopting a reasonable tone, she'd stall: "But look, I can tell you everything that's in the closet or anywhere else in the house. We've lived here fifteen years, me and you, remember?"

"So you've been snooping around my apartment. Now stop touching my things and get out before I call the cops."

In the early stages of the disease, Elizabeth had refused to give in. She went from room to room, holding up various knickknacks: a lamp they had found on Cape Cod that he insisted on buying because it was both elegant and ridiculous. "A bit of you and a bit of me," he joked when they brought it home.

But nothing she said did any good. He asked her to stop making up stories and then demanded that she stop bringing *her* stuff to *his* apartment.

The more desperate she sounded, the angrier he became, as if *he* was the one indulging a delusional person. Some evenings, he flew into a rage, grabbed her by the neck like a stray cat, and pushed her out the front door. And there she'd sit all night in the hallway.

But Mitch wasn't predictable—sometimes he seemed perfectly normal in the evenings; at other times, he magnanimously let her remain. But his episodes grew more frequent and his recalcitrance more extreme, and soon her exile in the hallway became almost a nightly routine. She took to carrying a spare key in her pocket and would let herself in when she thought Mitch had fallen asleep.

Telling me all this, Elizabeth added, "I wish I hadn't put the two of us through it."

"How was any of this your fault?" I asked.

"Oh, I could have stopped pleading and arguing with him much earlier. It would have saved us both a lot of heartache. It just took me so long to learn my lesson."

"I doubt it," I replied, knowing how many people never attain such distance.

But Elizabeth shook her head. "It's my biggest regret."

I asked her why she fell into the trap of arguing with Mitch when she knew she couldn't win.

She chuckled. "The thing is, he had an answer for everything. No matter what I said or could prove, he had an explanation. I just couldn't let it go."

Seeing my sympathetic expression, she said, "People

always ask about the patient. 'How is Mitch? How's he doing?' Let me tell you something, the patient is fine; it's the caregiver who's going crazy."

WHEN PATIENTS HAVE AN ANSWER for everything, caregivers get caught in a loop. It's surprisingly hard not to be goaded by a patient's responses. Even if the answers are nonsensical, the patient's ability to provide them suggests that we are still dealing with a functional mind. Indeed, that part of the mind which helps patients produce a steady stream of answers remains intact. It was this part—what the neuroscientist Michael Gazzaniga has termed the "left-brain interpreter"— that Mitch was now leaning on. The "interpreter" is an unconscious process responsible for sweeping inconsistencies and confusion under the rug. When things don't add up, when our expectations are flipped, when our environment surprises us, the left-brain interpreter provides explanations that help us make sense of things.

Although we rely on facts and logic in our daily lives, we tend to massage them when they fail to conform to our expectations. We saw this with the visual system. When our "visual interpreter" falls for optical illusions or smoothes over visual glitches, it does so in accordance with certain preconceptions. Similarly, our left-brain interpreter fills in cognitive blind spots, hiccups, ambiguities, and gaps.

But as useful as the "interpreter" is, it can also fail if "hijacked" by bad information. Bad information can come in various forms, both internal and external. For example, there is a bizarre condition that superficially resembles Mitch's case called Capgras syndrome. Capgras syndrome is a psychiatric disorder that causes people to think their loved ones are impostors or have been replaced by identical doubles. Capgras patients become enraged by people they know well because suddenly they appear to be malicious strangers. Mitch may not have believed that Elizabeth was an identical double, but he did believe that she was an impostor pretending to be his wife.

In Capgras patients, the parts of the brain responsible for identifying people are in conflict. When a healthy person sees her mother, the recognition of "Mom" feels like a single thing, whereas in actuality it is the product of various regions or subcommittees in the brain working together to create a picture of "Mom." We're not privy to these unconscious activities; we just feel a unified neural conglomeration that we understand as the person "Mom." But in Capgras patients, the visual system confirms that someone *looks* like Mom while the emotional system disagrees because the person does not *feel* like Mom. In order to make sense of these conflicting messages, the "hijacked" left-brain interpreter jumps in to create a coherent story—e.g., the person must be an impostor. And since we aren't aware of these mixed messages, we're left only with the interpreter's answers.

In a similar manner, patients feeling anxious or afraid because of memory loss or confusion will come up with explanations for their disorientation. They'll blame the aide for misplacing a purse or insist that people are conspiring against them. When they feel internal discord, their unconscious mind searches for an external source, and this source gives shape to their paranoia. So when Mitch was confronted by evidence that Elizabeth was his wife, which contradicted his impression that she was someone else, his left-brain interpreter found explanations for that evidence—for instance, that it had been planted in his apartment.

This is partly why so many patients are adept at coming up with quick (albeit wrong) answers and rationalizations for their warped views. Mixed signals may be the pathology, but the mind's propensity to create believable narratives is all too human.

In a 1962 study that would surely be considered unethical today, Stanley Schachter and Jerry Singer administered epinephrine to their subjects. Epinephrine, a synthetic hormone that narrows blood vessels, can produce anxiety, shakiness, and sweating. Some participants were then informed that they had been given a vitamin that had no side effects. The others were told that the pill could produce a racing heart, tremors, and flushing. Those who knew about the possible side effects immediately attributed their discomfort to the drug. Those unaware of possible side effects experienced agitation and blamed their environment, even thinking that the other participants were responsible.

We evidently have a tendency to find reasons for what disturbs us rather than remain in the dark. This need to ascertain cause and effect is yet another function of the left-brain interpreter, and it plays out in many ways. For example, we'll assign reasons to our feelings despite often not knowing their true cause. We'll twist facts, defend misconceptions, and opt to believe whatever makes sense of what's happening around us.

Sadly, caregivers like Elizabeth must contend with people who are simultaneously lucid and confused, impaired yet oddly nimble, themselves and yet not themselves. And much like their patients, such caregivers do not take this confusion lying down. After all, the healthy mind also abhors inconsistencies, contradictions, and ambiguity, which, of course, is what dementia disorders regularly throw at them. In effect, patient and caregiver are locked in a battle of left-brain interpreters, each one determined to fend off the chaos the other one represents.

Naturally, the cost to the caregiver can be significant, especially during the early stages of dementia, when patients have surprising cognitive resources to draw on. During one of their nightly "battles," Mitch made good on his threat to call the police. He dialed 911 and claimed that a strange woman was in his apartment. Elizabeth had meanwhile picked up the other phone and whispered urgently that her husband had dementia and there was no need to waste the police's time. Twenty minutes later, however, two cops arrived to find an incensed Mitch and a sobbing Elizabeth. At which point something totally unexpected happened.

"Mitch became Mitch again," Elizabeth told me.

"How so?" I asked.

"He suddenly remembered me, and then, as if nothing were wrong, he offered the police a beer. He even asked if they could stay awhile. Of course, they said they had to go."

"So they didn't do anything?"

"Well, they told him I was his wife and to take it easy and that sort of thing."

"And what did Mitch do?"

"He just said, 'No problem. Glad you dropped by.' And

after they left, he was okay. He even asked me if I wanted to go out for dinner, even though we'd eaten two hours ago."

After the police left, Elizabeth realized that social stimulation reminded Mitch of who she was. Human interaction had washed away the agitation in his body and the chaos in his mind (thus leaving the left-brain interpreter with no threat to interpret). And because Mitch seemed to know her when people were around, their friends initially didn't understand what Elizabeth was going through. This, in turn, made her worry that people thought she was exaggerating her husband's dementia, since he seemed so normal in company.

AT ONE OF OUR FIRST meetings, Elizabeth remembered a particularly harrowing confrontation. Instead of throwing her out, Mitch had suddenly relaxed and turned on the TV. He flipped through the channels but stopped at the opening credits to *Doctor Zhivago* and, hearing "Lara's Theme," reached for her hand.

"Imagine," she said to me, "we were holding hands."

I pictured them together, sitting on a couch, as romantic music filled the air—a scene that would be touching if I didn't consider what such moments did to her.

"I was like an abused woman," she told me, "always on edge. I never knew which side of him was going to come out."

It was the perpetuation of the sweet Mitch that kept her off balance. Because alongside the man who didn't recognize her was the man who might stroke her hair and ask how she put up with him. Alongside the man who threw her out the door was the man who made a video for their anniversary in which he confessed how lost he'd be without her. If that Mitch did not exist—if Elizabeth had had only the delusional Mitch to deal with—her left-brain interpreter would have had less to contend with. Instead, her brain was badgered by inconsistency and uncertainty.

When we think of Alzheimer's, we usually think of it as erasing the self. But what happens in most cases is that the self splinters into different selves, some we recognize, others we don't. As with memory, the self is not, as the philosopher Patricia Churchland phrased it, an "all or nothing affair." Instead, our concept of ourselves is distributed throughout the brain, making Alzheimer's more complicated than is generally believed. If the self is, in some sense, *already* fragmented, its gradual erosion can remain unnoticed behind the ebb and flow of a person's familiar personality. Cases, of course, vary. Quite often, Alzheimer's doesn't get rid of the self as much as it brings some parts to the fore.

Philosophers have always disagreed over what makes a coherent self from one moment to the next, and most have considered this question with a degree of remove. Caregivers don't have this luxury; the question of their loved one's identity affects them existentially. Whose hand are they holding? What, for instance, makes Mitch "Mitch" as he shifts from nice to mean, from recognizing his wife to perceiving her as an intruder? The question of selfhood involved in dementia disorders also poses an ethical problem. Should we, for example, approve a medical procedure that a patient would not have wanted in the past but is now unable to understand or make a decision about?

A few decades ago, the philosopher Derek Parfit devised

a thought experiment in which one person's cells are gradually replaced by another person's cells. At what point, he wondered, does one self end and another begin? When we truly register the shifting, amorphous nature of the self, we see that there is no magical "stuff" or essence that clearly defines a person. For a philosopher like Parfit, the question is not about a moment when Mitch stops being Mitch, because there was never a "real" Mitch to begin with. Philosophers may care about truth, about what logically can and cannot constitute identity, but our minds have more urgent priorities, namely maintaining a connection with other people.

For Elizabeth, Mitch was still Mitch. A loved one's identity isn't something that evaporates when change occurs. One reason for this may be our unconscious belief in what the psychologist Paul Bloom refers to as the "essential self." Early in our development we attribute to other people a permanent "deep-down self." And though our understanding of people becomes more complex as we grow older, our belief in a "true" or "real" self persists.*

When experimental philosophers, interested in how we define the self, asked participants to consider what happens when a hypothetical brain transplant affects a subject's physical abilities, skill set, intelligence, personality, and memory, most participants continued to believe that the subject's "true self" remained intact. Only in those cases where the subject began to behave in morally uncharacteristic ways—stealing,

---

* When I speak of an intuition about the "true self," I am not suggesting that it is an error in thinking. I am simply pointing out that such intuitions often influence how we view and react to people with dementia.

murdering, downloading child pornography, or engaging in other abhorrent behaviors—did participants conclude that the "true self" had been radically altered.

Bloom explains that we feel this way because we're more likely to associate the "good" qualities in people with their true selves—"good," of course, as defined by our own values. In this sense, another person's "true" self is an extension of what we hold dear. So if the essential self is intuitively equated with the moral self, then the cognitive problems attending dementia can seem peripheral. A change in personality may therefore not seem "deep enough" to redefine a husband or a father. The reason that Elizabeth kept arguing with Mitch is that she was appealing to the "real" Mitch, the "good" Mitch, the one "still in there," the one who, in the past, would have come to her aid.

FOR CAREGIVERS, THE IDEA OF a "real self" can be a double-edged sword. If, on the one hand, it encourages us to argue with afflicted loved ones in the hope of breaking through to their "real selves," it can be a source of great frustration. If, on the other hand, we start to doubt the existence of an essential self, how can we account for the person we're caring for? Who is it that we are suffering and sacrificing for?

Seeing continuity in people is entirely natural and, real or not, the idea of an essential self has valuable, even practical applications. If we weren't built to believe that other people have essential selves, it would be too easy to become disconnected from family and friends. This is especially true if someone close to us sustains a head trauma or develops a disorder in the brain. And even when patients in the late stages of dementia disorder no longer recognize their families—or even themselves—caregivers maintain an unshakable feeling that they are still there, that despite everything they continue to be "Mom" and "Dad."

What about someone who changes for the better?

I spoke to one woman who had married a man who was gruff, surly, and mean-spirited. Perpetually dissatisfied, he assumed the worst of people and treated them accordingly. But when he developed frontotemporal dementia, his mood lightened. He became openly affectionate with his wife in public, both pleasing and embarrassing her. He began chatting and joking with the doormen he had formerly ignored or criticized. His memory compromised, he stopped working, but he also stopped holding grudges, and whatever bothered him was soon forgotten.

I don't often hear this kind of story, but when I do I'm glad for caregivers whose relationships, despite all the difficulties, become in some way easier. Nonetheless, I wondered what this woman felt when she walked and talked and slept with her husband. Did she ever feel that she was eating breakfast with a nice stranger? It was more likely that she felt she was eating with her newly nice husband. Our essentialist nature runs so deep that it's almost absurd to think about her situation in any other way.

The left-brain interpreter dismisses anomalies and weirdness and creates continuity even when the facts don't support it. Unlike the victims of Capgras syndrome, who see a familiar person but emotionally register a stranger, the rest of us seem determined to overlook the increasing strangeness of loved ones and continue to see an essential self.

NOWADAYS, MITCH IS MUCH CALMER—his confusion has ebbed along with his cognitive capacity—and so is Elizabeth. Even so, at our last meeting, Elizabeth told me that he can still, on occasion, become upset. One day when Mitch was filling in a coloring book, something he previously would have found beneath him, he looked up and said, "I think there's something wrong with me."

"Well, honey," Elizabeth said gently, "you have something called Alzheimer's, and that's okay, I'm here for you."

Mitch furrowed his brow. "No, that's not it. I don't have that. Why would you even say that?"

Elizabeth immediately retreated from the statement. "I felt awful getting him agitated like that," she told me.

"It's hard to resist," I said. "You were trying to give your husband permission to feel confusion by explaining the source."

"Yes," she said, "that's true. But you're giving me too much credit. I just wanted him to *get it,* so *both* of us would know. So we could be in on it together."

I nodded. For a moment, she believed she had glimpsed the old Mitch, the true Mitch, so she had confided in him, the way she had in the past, thinking he'd understand. But the moment passed, and she reprimanded herself for forgetting the lessons the disease had taught her. As she talked about it, her eyes began to well up, and I thought she was going to acknowledge, as so many caregivers do, how hard and lonely it was to take care of her husband, how there was a part of her that wished it would end.

What she said took me aback.

"You know, I'm very grateful for this experience in a way. Don't get me wrong, it's a terrible disease and I wouldn't wish it on anyone. But I've learned a lot about myself. I've learned about my limitations, and I guess I've learned I can survive. I have more patience than I thought. I didn't expect to, but I've learned there's still love, and love doesn't go away. Alzheimer's can't take it away. And so I feel grateful."

I was moved, as I often am when I hear about the redemptive aspects of caregiving. Then I surprised myself by adding that she must have felt very different during the early stages of the disease.

"Oh, God, yes," she said.

After she left, I wondered why I had reminded her of those painful days when she found herself sitting in the hallway outside her apartment, furious and devastated that Mitch didn't know her. I realized it came from a misplaced sense of protectiveness toward her. Apparently I was still stuck on her suffering. Knowing everything that she had gone through, I wasn't ready to let Alzheimer's off the hook. The disease didn't deserve her tolerance or gratitude. In a way, I was trying to square my own sense of who she was. After all, the composed woman who had just left my office was no longer the woman who had been exiled from her home.

According to Kahneman, there are indeed two different Elizabeths: the person who experienced an event and the person who remembers it, and each one measures pain differently. The "experiencing self" is, of course, transient; the "remembering self" persists; it continues to modulate experience (in left-brain-interpreter mode), building a neater, more coherent narrative. Elizabeth's early caregiving days and Mitch's obstreperous behavior were now being massaged by her remembering self. This allowed Elizabeth to tease from events a meaning that hadn't been there for the experiencing self.

Kahneman's two selves can make interviewing caregivers a tricky proposition. People actively invested in caregiving may have neither the time nor the inclination to talk to me, while those finished with caregiving often have difficulty recalling the specifics of the painful events they lived through. When these veteran caregivers sit down to talk, they seem more intent on imparting the important lessons they've learned than on recalling what actually happened and how it made them feel. They're not deliberately withholding facts; it's just that once the emotional turmoil has died down, the remembering self takes over, weaving redemptive lessons into a more linear, comprehensible narrative.

When I walked home after seeing Elizabeth for the last time, I was still mulling over my preoccupation with the "experiencing" Elizabeth I'd first met rather than the resilient woman she had become. And it occurred to me that my resistance to Elizabeth's sense of contentment was the same resistance I felt to the ending of one of my favorite plays, Chekhov's *Uncle Vanya*. In the final scene, Sonya and Vanya suffer from unrequited love and pangs of remorse. By now

Uncle Vanya has realized that his mentor, Professor Sere-bryakov, whom he had faithfully served for so many years, is a charlatan, unworthy of his affection and loyalty.

As the sounds of crickets fill the air, Vanya and Sonya return to work, retreating into the minutiae that have defined and diminished their lives. After a moment, Vanya glances up from Serebryakov's papers and admits to feeling despondent. But instead of the play ending on a quiet note of resignation, Sonya delivers a hysterically hopeful speech: "We shall rejoice and look back at our present misfortunes with a feeling of tenderness, with a smile—we shall rest, we shall rest. I believe, Uncle, I believe in it fervently and passionately."

This outburst rang false to me. Chekhov's characters have good reason to suffer. So why inject the ending with unearned hope?

It then occurred to me that Chekhov simply understood that while we can endure the most painful heartbreak or terrible disappointment, we cannot live with the idea that such experiences have no meaning. Sonya, in fact, is like many caregivers who look back on their struggles with a "feeling of tenderness," healing themselves by reconfiguring a painful experience. When Elizabeth considered the turmoil she had endured, she felt that it had only reinforced her love for Mitch.

Dementia disorders may bring chaos, devastation, and loss, but the mind is not without its defenses. It continues to weave a meaningful narrative, even from events that threaten to diminish essential parts of our loved ones and ourselves.

5

The Insistent, Persistent CEO

Why We Feel Patients Are Still Capable of Self-Awareness

AS A CHILD GROWING UP IN RED HOOK, BROOKLYN, LANI FALCO dreaded going home. She preferred the action on the streets—docks where men in work clothes shambled back and forth, or the stoops of row houses where loud women in curlers gossiped and smoked, or street corners where a group of men stood together talking and gesticulating, falling silent whenever she approached. Although nothing much ever happened, she had the sense that at least something *could* happen. But within the four rooms of the federal housing project that she shared with her mother, two younger sisters, and autistic brother, she expected nothing but noise. Her mother,

Tina—stressed and addled—only compounded the clamor from which Lani desperately wanted to escape.

At eighteen, she did exactly that. She took a job as a bartender near the Brooklyn courthouse. It wasn't a yuppie bar but a neighborhood haunt where she bantered with sharpies and crooks along with high-powered lawyers, judges, and journalists. For Lani the bar was a magical place where the currency was not money or power but stories. Every night she watched people trickle in, anticipating the play that was about to begin; she was rarely disappointed. Tending bar, she received news of the world; in Red Hook, the news was always the same.

I got to know Lani in the fall of 2016. Although we'd spoken over the phone a few times, I didn't expect the long, wavy, reddish hair or the flowing vintage dress and cowboy boots. We met at her local bakery and, as promised, she wore a flower in her hair. When I spotted it and walked over, she jumped up, gave me a big hug, and insisted I try her biscotti. It took all of sixty seconds to learn that she was a pleasing mix of warmth and bluntness. Quick, smart, and self-educated, Lani would pick up a book whenever she had a free moment, any book as long as it was serious: social science, history, biography, and especially philosophy.

On Sundays, Lani visited her mother. Tina had developed Alzheimer's two years earlier and, over her objections, Lani had managed to install a live-in aide, a capable Jamaican woman named Amoy. Tina alternately resented Amoy, relied on her, and forgot she existed. She was becoming more and more bull-headed as the disease progressed, and Lani wasn't keen on visiting. Nonetheless, every Sunday she went back to Red Hook.

When Tina was diagnosed, Lani began researching the disease. She read as much as she could, including a good deal of the medical literature. So when she fought with Tina, it wasn't lost on her that she was "not picking on someone my own size."

"The thing you need to know about my mom," she told me that day in the bakery, "is that she always chooses the dumbest, hardest, most ass-backwards path, then defends it and suffers the consequences."

It was the trajectory of this path that both saddened and frustrated Lani. Tina was a child of the Depression who had lost her own mother at ten and was forced to care for her siblings while her father, a bricklayer, scrounged to put food on the table. Life was hard, and her siblings resented Tina for overseeing them. It wasn't long after she had finished raising them that she had kids of her own.

Lani's father had been a decent man, religious and unimaginative. He read the Bible, didn't care for socializing, and worked long hours. He'd been an administrator on the docks, dealing with bills of lading and transfers of freight. Growing up, Lani sensed that whatever passion had driven her parents to marry had dissipated long ago. When Lani was sixteen, her father suffered a hemorrhagic stroke and died a few days later. And Tina, who had always been anxious, now concentrated on just making ends meet.

Even as a child, Lani was disturbed by her mother's refusal to acknowledge reality. Tina refused help and rarely slept, and the more exhausted she became, the more responsibility she took on herself—all the while denying that anything was wrong. Later, when Lani urged her to see a therapist, Tina scoffed. Stress only made her more determined to push through. But her resulting exhaustion led her to make poor choices, even around the medical care for her autistic son.

Alzheimer's further skewed the picture, and for Tina the diagnosis became something else to doggedly overcome. Every day, she organized and reorganized the kitchen, taking items from one spot, putting them somewhere else, and then forgetting what she'd done. And when she couldn't find something, she blamed Amoy. Sometimes, convinced that her son, Bobby, who still lived with her, wanted a grilled cheese and tomato sandwich, she'd start making it, forget what she was doing, and start over again. Lani might arrive home to find her mother exhausted and disoriented, with ten or twelve half-made sandwiches spread around the kitchen.

Naturally, Lani begged her mother to stop and relax, but Tina didn't know how. Her habit of controlling the chaos in her life turned to frenzy as her Alzheimer's worsened. Here was a woman, Lani told me, who required total control but was now constantly reminded that she had none. A woman who had always needed to be right suddenly found herself coping with a disease that made her feel like a screw-up.

Feeling compassion for Tina, however, didn't help Lani deal with her mother's symptoms. Prone to dehydration, Tina was supposed to drink four or five glasses of water a day, but when Amoy tried to hand her a glass, Tina would wave her away. She refused to do almost anything Amoy suggested, because it would mean caving in or losing control. This meant that Lani often received Amoy's frantic middle-of-the-night phone calls from the emergency room when Tina was admitted with dehydration.

Talking to Tina about any of this did no good. She'd simply look aggrieved, as though she was the victim of a great injustice. Asked to change her behavior and listen to Amoy, Tina would nod but refuse to engage. The same passivity that Lani had always met with continued after Tina's diagnosis. Whatever accusations Lani threw at her, whatever opinions she expressed, whatever help she offered were all met with the same indifference.

If Lani said, as she sometimes did, "Because you don't listen, I'm losing money. I'm always here instead of working," her mother simply looked off into the distance and mumbled, "If she had a normal office job, she'd be much better off. But no, she chose to make a career of pouring drinks."

Usually Lani ignored such comments, but one day, she lost her temper: "Damn it, Ma, what the hell does that have to do with anything?"

To this, her mother calmly responded: "Okay, Lani. You know everything, you always did."

Telling me this, Lani started to laugh. Tina had managed to deflect criticism of herself and redirect it toward her daughter. And it worked. Instead of frightening Tina, Lani managed only to scare herself. Although Tina's criticism had not bothered her in the past, it now hit a nerve.

Five years earlier Lani had started a business restoring old furniture, but just as her new career was getting off the ground, Tina had been diagnosed and soon required all the attention and energy that should have gone into the shop. Taking care of Tina, interceding between her and Amoy, and fretfully waiting for the phone to ring drained Lani completely.

Every argument, every unscheduled trip home, every fearful trip to the emergency room made her feel as though her life—and her mind—were slipping away. Increasingly she felt herself mirroring her mother's cognitive issues: her forgetfulness, her inability to focus, her poor judgment.

"I'M A SELFISH PERSON," LANI told me at our second meeting. She had come to my office late one afternoon, bringing along a loaf of bread that she had baked. After we cut ourselves slices, she said, "I don't want to be a martyr. I'll never forgive myself if I let her take over my life."

I nodded but sensed that what she really meant was that she did not want to become her mother—not just the Tina of today but the Tina of her childhood, a woman so dulled by the burdens of being a wife and mother that she had no curiosity, no energy, no life force to engage the world. And it was this fear that occasionally made Lani lash out. She had started to pick fights with Tina, provoking her even when she was napping or doing nothing, quiet moments that Lani usually relished.

"Why do you think you do it?" I asked.

"I'm just a dog with a bone," she said. Then she took a moment to consider. "I don't know—maybe it's because it's a way of separating myself from Mom's life."

By now such insights from Lani didn't surprise me.

"Let me tell you what I did the other day," she said. "I startled her awake and then told her for the hundredth time that she had to listen to Amoy, that I wanted her to be safe. So she said the doctors told her she was fine. *That* she remembers. So I said the doctors were just being nice, they want to make her feel good. Then I joked, 'Luckily you have me.' You know, she chuckled at that. I should have stopped there, but of course I continued to poke. So I said, 'Remember what *else* they told you? They said you're dangerously dehydrated, which means you have to drink water when Amoy gives it to you. You have to listen to her.'"

She paused, as though remembering.

"Then what happened?" I asked.

"Oh, the usual. When she's backed into a corner and realizes she's run out of excuses, she plays the victim and starts to whine. 'You don't understand what it's like,' she says. And I say something like 'I understand that you need help'— which gets her angry and she tells me in her usual superior tone that I'm the one who doesn't understand, that I understand nothing, that I just go around telling people what to do."

As Lani spoke, I felt her frustration spiking.

"Anyway, this time I couldn't take it anymore," she said. "Enough was enough. So I got in her face and said, 'No, *you* don't understand! You have dementia! You want everyone to suffer because you can't accept that you have a problem. Remember how many times we went to the emergency room just because you didn't listen?' And what does my mom say? She looks off somewhere and repeats the usual, 'Yeah, yeah. You know everything, you always did.'"

To an outsider, this exchange might seem cruel. Why confront Tina with her own helplessness? But frustrated caregivers often refute patients' illusions of independence, not only because they're angry but also because some part of them believes that the patient is still in charge. By demanding that Tina cede control, Lani was laboring under the illusion that her mother had enough awareness to know what was happening to her. It's an assumption that consciousness instills in us.

Consciousness may be the ultimate lottery prize of evolution, allowing us to adapt and change as our environment changes, but it is also quite capable of deluding itself. As Michael Gazzaniga explains in *Who's in Charge? Free Will and the Science of the Brain,* consciousness in human beings is accompanied by the intuition that we have volition and free will. And this intuition is continually reinforced by the story consciousness invents, the one in which consciousness is responsible for all our actions. It's why people who are not in control continue to act as though they are.

The neuroscientist David Eagleman takes this assessment a step further, comparing consciousness to the CEO of a big company who believes they're running things but often has no idea what's going on or what is actually required to make the company function smoothly. Like CEOs who credit themselves for their company's performance, consciousness assumes it's the orchestrator of thoughts and actions even though it remains completely unaware of the enormous unconscious input of what Eagleman calls the brain's various "subcommittees." Although much of our decision-making stems from Kahneman's System 1's automatic unconscious processing, it's the "CEO," or System 2, that insists that it's in charge. Which makes sense, since thoughts and actions *should* feel like they're coming from the conscious, in-charge "Me."

In 1983 the neuroscientist Benjamin Libet measured

consciousness's role in behavior. He placed electrodes on participants' heads and instructed them to lift a finger when they felt like it. A curious thing happened: The electroencephalogram (EEG) recorded that participants felt motivated to lift the finger before they were conscious of their willingness to do so. In other words, the unconscious subunits in the brain make decisions before we're actually aware of them. Consciousness may feel in charge, but sometimes it's just playing catch-up to what our unconscious system has already decided.*

The feeling that we control our behavior aligns with the general intuition that intention precedes action. But does it? The social psychologist Daniel M. Wegner and others contend that the sensation of consciously willing something to happen is "the mind's best trick." In one well-known experiment, scientists attempted to measure the degree to which people think they control their own behavior. Participants sat in front of a screen with hands outstretched. They were told that when the screen turned red they should choose one hand to raise, either the right or the left, but not to raise it until the screen turned green. After red, the screen turned yellow, then green, at which point the participants lifted the hand they had chosen.

Next the participants were given the same instructions,

---

* The empirical measurement of consciousness is still in its infancy and the debate regarding the conclusions drawn from such experiments has hardly died down. My references to these experiments neither affirm nor dismiss the role of "consciousness," "free will," or "self-control." And while some researchers believe that consciousness itself is an illusion, other researchers (including Libet) disagree. My purpose here is to reveal how the mind tends to view itself rather than to make any definitive claims *about* the mind.

but this time when the yellow screen appeared, a transcranial magnetic stimulation (TMS) sent a magnetic pulse to either the left or right side of the motor cortex, which made participants favor one hand over the other. Nonetheless, participants reported that they had chosen which hand they raised. In other words, consciousness is so greedy for control that it feels ownership for decisions it does not make.

This overestimation of the role of consciousness applies not only to small decisions but also to decisions that have real-life consequences. When judges, for instance, justify their verdicts, they believe their deliberations issue from moral reasoning or from objective legal analyses. If informed that hunger pangs, implicit racist biases, crankiness, or general human fallibility plays a part in their decisions (often taking the form of more conservative and punitive verdicts), they would undoubtedly and hotly dispute the imputation.

Consciousness may be the last to know why we act in certain ways, but it is the first to take credit. Moreover, it's "expensive," since, as previously noted, conscious processes use more energy than unconscious processes. Nonetheless, like the CEO of a big company, it's an essential expense, because despite its failings, consciousness plays a crucial role in mediating conflict between our unconscious processes. Without it we would have no cognitive flexibility, since consciousness would not be there to step in when things go awry.

In the "healthy brain," the CEO can relax, blithely letting unconscious processes do most of the work. But in the brain that is beginning to break down, Eagleman's CEO analogy takes on a certain poignancy. Despite glitches and memory loss, the CEO doesn't suddenly resign. It continues to assure everyone, especially itself, that it's still in charge. And like a typical CEO, it blames others for what goes wrong.

To people suffering from a dementia disorder, their problems are usually someone else's fault. If one of the jobs of consciousness is to run interference when there is a hiccup in perception or recognition, then the dementia patient's "CEO" must constantly intervene as the brain's subcommittees grow less and less proficient. So when dementia patients put the teakettle in the microwave or the laundry detergent in the oven, the CEO is called in to do damage control. When Tina, for example, positioned the knives in a drawer so that the blades faced dangerously outward, it was because "this way I can see what I have and if anyone took anything."

CAREGIVERS THUS CONTEND WITH A dual problem: Although they know what the disease does, they often believe their loved ones remain in charge despite evidence to the contrary. It's this evidence—the symptoms themselves—that summons the addled patient's CEO. It wasn't the glitches in Tina's zombie systems that frustrated Lani; it was the meddling CEO hovering, rationalizing, and blaming others. And the more Tina's CEO micromanaged and deflected from her internal chaos, the easier it was for both Tina and Lani to misjudge the extent of the disease's encroachment. Of course, it didn't help that Tina's CEO mimicked her usual managerial style ("Sure, Lani, you know everything"). All of which made it easier for Lani to think that her mother still knew what she was doing.

How much simpler life would be if the patient's CEO

stepped aside in a timely manner, recognizing that they could no longer function effectively. Were this to happen, the disease would be laid bare. But because the CEO covers up with familiar behavior, a caregiver is pulled into a patient's illusion of self-awareness. And this illusion is bolstered by the patient's occasional lucid moments.

When Tina said, "I know that of all people, you won't sugarcoat things. Am I going crazy?," it broke Lani's heart to see her mother so vulnerable. So she quickly assured Tina that she wasn't crazy, she just had "a touch of dementia" and that she, Lani, was taking care of things. Although these moments of self-awareness were sporadic, they made Lani think that deep down her mother understood her predicament and was simply *choosing,* as she had always done, to deny reality and make things harder for everyone around her.

Moreover, consciousness is not only less omniscient than it believes, it's also not just one thing. The brain is composed, as Gazzaniga has shown, of plural, localized consciousnesses. There is no singular CEO, no one boss who calls the shots. (Eagleman's CEO is, of course, just an allegorical device.) If consciousness were just one entity or function, a severe injury or neurological condition like Alzheimer's would destroy it. But consciousness is too important to be stored in one place. Instead, it's distributed in different localities, so it has backup systems to protect it. If consciousness existed in only a single location, all the neurons in the brain would have to be synchronized, and it would take more time—and energy—for information to reach that one destination. The decentralized brain is thus more secure and more efficient.

So even when people fall prey to dementia, consciousness is safeguarded. Moreover, the left-brain interpreter is still weaving singular story lines that make sense of the brain's competing, buzzing subunits. Patients continue to see themselves as a unified self, and this is the self, however impaired, that a patient presents to the world. To Lani, Tina seemed like a person who simply chose when to acknowledge her disease and when to deny it.

LANI, BEING LANI, WAS FAMILIAR with Michael Gazzaniga's *Who's in Charge?* She understood why the mind is predisposed to feel in charge and that the feeling is often an illusion. She knew that we tend to overestimate the conscious "I," attributing to it a volition it doesn't always possess. She also appreciated the fact that a "deep-down self" might be a figment or, at best, a much more complex and fragmented sort of self.

But no matter how much she engaged with these ideas intellectually, Lani the thinker was different from Lani the daughter. When she engaged with her mother, all bets were off. Alzheimer's or no Alzheimer's, she couldn't see Tina as a damaged cortex or a body without a watchful mind, and she reacted to Tina's personality and actions as she always had.

"Everything I tell the aide not to do," Lani said ruefully, "I do myself. When Amoy and I talk on the phone, I tell her that arguing with my mom is like arguing with cancer. You can't talk it away. You're arguing with a broken machine, not a mind. 'There's no there there,' I tell her. But then I go over on Sundays and I'm no different. I get involved in all this arguing and screaming. Jesus, I feel like such a hypocrite."

When she said this, I told her what I tell all caregivers: "When it comes to dementia disorders, we're all hypocrites at one time or another."

Lani gave me one of her big, warm smiles. She thought I was trying to excuse her "bad" behavior. But that's not what I was doing, not exactly. I was simply normalizing her behavior.

In *Descartes' Baby*, Paul Bloom reveals that human beings are born dualist, treating the mind and body as separate entities. Even when adults understand how the brain works, their intuition tells them that some aspect of the mind—call it an essence or spirit—cannot be reduced to a neurological mechanism. It's a default stance found across cultures.*

What caregivers are constantly told to do is to regard a patient's wants, demands, and intentions as issuing from an impaired brain, not from a mind in charge of itself. Friends, family, and health professionals all remind us: "It's not them, it's their brain. They can't help it." Yet in case after case, in family after family, caregivers like Lani who know better continue to react to the disease as though its victims are still in control.

Caregivers are not alone in this error. Doctors, scientists, even hard-nosed neuroscientists often turn out to be "card-carrying dualists." Sure, it's easy for people to say, "Your mom is not doing anything on purpose, she has a disease," but

---

* The mind-body problem endures. Many philosophers believe the mind to be nothing more than the product of the brain's activities. Other philosophers believe this to be a reductive position that overlooks important issues such as qualia (i.e., subjective aspects of our mental life). Here, as elsewhere, I do not take a stand on the matter. As I do with other human intuitions and proclivities, I refer to "dualism" only insofar as it colors our view of people with dementia.

should *their* spouse or parent develop a dementia disorder, they too will occasionally feel that the patient's aggravating behaviors issue from a willful mind, not a diseased brain. The reason dualism persists is that, at bottom, the mind-body distinction isn't theoretical, it's *biological*. We cannot get rid of this intuition even if we wanted to; it's part of our cognitive architecture.

AS LANI SPOKE TO ME about the existence of free will and the nature of consciousness and identity, her words poured out with increasing urgency, trying to keep up with her thoughts. What bothered her was her inability to distinguish between the disease and her mother even though she knew—knew for certain—that Tina's brain was impaired.

"I don't know where to draw the line," she said. "Do you?"

I thought for a moment and then asked if the question itself wasn't misleading.

"How do you mean?" she asked, a gleam in her eye.

"Well, perhaps the question already presumes a duality. It presumes that there's still a 'ghost in the machine'"—a term coined by the Oxford philosopher Gilbert Ryle that casts doubt on the Cartesian division between mind and body. The ghost here is not the mind but rather mental activity in general, as distinct from the body or any physical activity.

Lani, already familiar with the phrase, was right there with me. "So you're saying the same thing, right? There is no line."

"Yes—but even talking about a line," I said, "kind of defeats the purpose of trying to say there isn't one. As long as we say there's a line where the disease begins and the person ends, aren't we still suggesting that dementia disorders affect one and not the other—and that a special part of ourselves somehow remains immune?"

I stopped, suddenly feeling self-conscious. "I'm no different from anyone else. Nobody really gets away from the dualism."*

Lani chuckled. "You don't have to coddle me. I love this stuff. I need juice, you know? I need someone to argue with. Talk things out with. It helps me understand what I'm thinking and whether I'm full of it, which I usually am."

She was being too hard on herself. Everyone Lani had grown up with, including her mother, thought she was a know-it-all, but Lani simply *wanted* to know it all, which is why she encouraged me to challenge her as she jumped from one idea to another. Wasn't it, then, both ironic and redemptive that her mother's dementia had brought her to a place where suddenly ideas weren't abstractions? Now she could ponder philosophical concepts *and* know them in a way that was not academic: Who is Tina now that her brain is being altered by dementia? What defines identity? What is the nature of consciousness?

Whether caregivers know about Cartesian dualism or not, they still have to reject it every day in order to deal effectively with family members who have become patients. Somehow they're supposed to overcome a philosophical conundrum that has confounded thinkers for nearly two millennia. And even more improbably, they are expected to do it alone.

---

* Again, this is not a rebuttal of dualism but rather a comment on how powerful this intuition is.

6

When Every Day Is Sunday

Why We Dispute a Patient's Reality

AT THE OUTSET OF MY FIRST INTERVIEW WITH CATHY O'BRIEN IN the winter of 2016, she cautioned, "You should know, I'm not a saint."

I assured her I didn't know any caregivers who were, nor did I want to meet any.

"That's good," she said.

Cathy is petite, in her late sixties, with short-cropped, shiny gray hair and a warm, tremulous voice. For six years, she had been taking care of her husband, Frank, but had recently started berating herself for not being "cut from the same cloth as Mother Teresa."

Frank, she told me, had always been the more religiously

conservative one, and when he developed Alzheimer's his Catholicism became more pronounced. Prior to the disease, he'd had a healthy dose of skepticism, something they had in common. But as his memory began to fail, the prudish, rule-bound side of him emerged. Dementia, Cathy said wryly, had brought out his "inner Catholic boy."

Watching her husband become more religious was both infuriating and alienating. Frank began to fixate on ritual, insisting they attend church every Sunday. This would have been fine, but for Frank, every day was Sunday. Every few hours he'd urge Cathy to get dressed and accompany him to church. Cathy would point out that it was a Wednesday or a Saturday, but Frank wouldn't be put off. She'd show him a calendar or a newspaper, and he would be mollified for a while. But then he'd forget and again tell her to get dressed. The only way Cathy could make it stick was to call the priest and ask him to reassure Frank.

"What do you do when your husband takes a priest's word over your own?" I asked.

She chuckled. "Well, I get angry, even though it doesn't really surprise me. Frank always had a thing for authority figures. He believes in them."

What irked Cathy even more than Frank's not believing her, or his hanging on to the priest's every word, was how he wore his piety on his sleeve. Watching him slowly cross himself in church made Cathy want to smack the righteous look off his face. "It's like being married to the pope," she said.

It's not uncommon for people with Alzheimer's to turn to religion. Because the disease routinely triggers the attachment system, patients—in addition to fixating on their parents or childhood homes—often take comfort in religion, another "safe base." They compensate for their illness and vulnerability with a kind of extreme piety that makes it hard to see the disease. When Cathy watched him in church, his mind steadied by his environment, he seemed in his element. Yet she also felt that he was "showing off," making a point of being righteous, especially in front of the priest. Although she knew that this was his way of self-soothing, of dealing with memory loss and confusion, she felt stifled by his overly earnest, at times cartoonish behavior.

As the disease progressed, Frank gradually stopped seeing Cathy as a complete person. She became a prop, a vessel into which he poured his fixations. So while Frank was able to sublimate his internal chaos by turning to ritual, Cathy had no one and nothing to turn to. Instead she found herself living with a humorless stranger.

It wasn't only his religiosity that narrowed her existence. Frank had taken to watching TV all day long. The first thing he did in the afternoon was grab the remote, plant himself in his favorite chair, and turn on a game. If it wasn't the Mets, it was the Jets. If it wasn't the Jets, it was the Rangers or the Knicks or the Giants. And he was not a passive spectator. He behaved as if he were sitting next to the dugout so the players would know what he thought when someone fumbled a ground ball or missed a tag. In fact, he began to excitedly predict when someone would screw up. "Don't do it!" he'd yell. "Wait! Wait!"

Movies also agitated him. He would yell at the actors, warning them of some impending disaster. Or he'd forecast some dire plot twist, shaking his fist at the TV. And if an attractive actress showed up, he might suddenly shout, "That woman is about to take her top off! No one wants to see that!" His impromptu yelling and ridiculous predictions sucked the joy out of everything.

One evening, after a few months of this, Cathy abruptly stood up and escaped to the bathroom.

"I couldn't sit there and keep my mouth shut, but I didn't want to argue with him," Cathy told me. "So I went off where I could scream."

Standing at the bathroom mirror, she saw an exhausted woman whose blank expression made her seem detached from reality. There and then she made a pact with her reflection: She'd leave Frank. She'd done her bit, and now she deserved a life of her own—a life without religious observance and constant yelling. Giving herself permission to leave calmed her down. She washed her face and took a few deep breaths, but walking back to the living room felt like walking to her death.

"Know what made it even worse?" she asked. "As soon as he saw me, his face broke into a huge smile. God, he's always so happy when he sees me, telling me how much he loves me even though he barely knows who I am anymore. But I can't bring myself to say it back. What's wrong with me? Shouldn't I want to be with him, take care of him?

"Of course I should. He's sick. He has a disease," she answered herself. "I should be able to take his yelling and his stupid predictions. Instead, I correct him. I tell him Errol Flynn isn't going to die. I tell him Doris Day isn't going to take her blouse off. Why do I do that? I mean, what do I care what the hell he says?"

She gave me a bashful look. "You know, there are times I still tell him it's Wednesday when he thinks it's Friday. I mean, that's Alzheimer's 101; you don't do that."

I smiled and said that I wished I could count the number of caregivers who have done more or less the same thing.

She harrumphed her solidarity with them. "You know, if someone had told me before Frank got Alzheimer's that all I had to do was agree with him and accept his reality, I would have said, 'Sure, what's so hard about that?' Who cares that he thinks some jock is going to fall on his ass or that the weather girl is going to flash everyone? I should let it go. It's not his fault."

Nor is it Cathy's fault. Human beings are "ultra-social" animals who require other people to see the world as they do. This need for a shared reality not only creates a connection to others but also validates feelings, judgments, and sense of self. Without such validation, we become both physically agitated and cognitively uncertain about what we know and who we are. Moreover, this need for a mutually agreed-upon reality is so strong that we naturally overestimate the degree to which others, especially loved ones, share our thoughts and perceptions. So when a spouse or parent suddenly sees the world very differently from us, we might intellectually register this as a symptom but unconsciously feel that an implicit social promise has been broken.

OVER THE COURSE OF MY meetings with Cathy, Frank began to develop new symptoms. He became convinced that thieves were staking out the house. He insisted on locking the doors and closing the windows come rain or shine. His frequent warnings and excessive vigilance made Cathy increasingly claustrophobic.

She put up with his delusions for months until one day she simply snapped. "No one is out to get you!" she shouted. "No one wants anything from you. You have dementia! Dementia!"

But to Frank, only the threat of being robbed was real; his dementia was not. "What are you doing to me?" he retorted. "What's wrong with *you*?"

Recounting this to me, Cathy shook her head in disbelief. "You know, he's absolutely right. I don't know what's wrong with me. I don't blame him for getting angry. If someone told me I had dementia, I'd hate it. So why do I act like this? Who does this?"

This ill-tempered side of herself was hard for Cathy to accept. "I always thought I was a sensitive person," she said. "Now I've become someone who kicks people when they're down."

Although she resented Frank for not understanding what the disease was doing to him, Cathy did not truly appreciate what the disease was doing to *her*. Dementia affects emotional regulation, so while we naturally expect patients to "lose it" every so often, we expect ourselves to keep it together. At first blush this makes sense. Unlike the impaired brain, the healthy brain has an intact prefrontal cortex (PFC), where self-regulation takes place. Nonetheless, this is no guarantee that we can always self-regulate.

Scientists have identified two kinds of regulation strategies in the PFC: automatic and effortful. Self-regulation is effortful when we experience a threat alone: More energy is then required to de-escalate emotions like anger and sadness. Solitary self-regulation, in fact, is meant to be draining, since we have evolved to co-regulate one another. Co-regulation, on the other hand, is automatic. In fact, the neurological divide between our stress and someone else's stress is not clearly delineated. Indeed, in some cases we seem to encode threats against others as we would against ourselves.

The brain's tendency to experience threats communally is part of what psychologists call *load sharing*. As its name suggests, load sharing is a way of conserving energy by de-escalating anxiety and stress. At some point in our evolution, load sharing became an adaptive mechanism to keep people close not only because there is safety in numbers, but also because threats feel less overwhelming in a community.

Hence, people in healthy and supportive relationships feel threats less intensely than people who feel alone. But that doesn't mean that a relationship is necessarily beneficial. If, like Cathy, we're technically not alone but *feel* alone, self-regulation becomes effortful. Is it any wonder that dementia caregivers struggle to keep their anger in check?

Consider what happens when a spouse or relative gets cancer: Patient and caregiver can commiserate, acknowledging the miseries of the disease while experiencing, to some degree, the reality of it together. Dementia, however, usually precludes the possibility of co-regulation. Patients often do not know—or resist knowing—that they have a neurological illness and, through no fault of their own, retreat to a world where caregivers cannot follow. While caregivers can certainly sense the stress that dementia patients feel, patients rarely grasp what caregivers are going through. So who is there to co-regulate the caregivers? The sad truth is that most caregivers end up feeling alone; and with no one to validate the burden of their reality, they may become as volatile as the people they care for.

AFTER CATHY HAD TAKEN CARE of Frank for about six years, the unfairness of it all began to weigh on her. She hated being stuck at home and hated herself for feeling that way.

Despite everything she did to make him feel safe, Frank still refused to crack a window, wary of imaginary thieves. "Okay, of course I get it," she told me. "I mean the poor guy is riddled with delusions. He has hallucinations. But I do everything for him, and I can't even get a little fresh air. I get so angry about how unfair it is, and then I feel so petty and selfish for feeling this way."

Cathy's reaction was understandable. Unfairness is not really about getting your own way—it's not about a shut window, it's not about who does the dishes. Unfairness marks a loss of social connection, a feeling that one more implicit social agreement has been canceled.

According to the social psychologist Matthew D. Lieberman, fairness not only feels right, it also registers in the brain as deeply pleasurable. Fairness, he writes, "tastes like chocolate." Perhaps if I had less experience with caregivers, that line might have struck me as an amusing exaggeration. Instead it brought to mind someone in one of my support groups who, in trying to describe the lack of emotional reciprocity between her and her husband, blurted out, "I feel that I'm starving. I think we're all starving."

The group knew immediately what she meant. There is nothing fair about a long-standing relationship suddenly becoming one-sided. It isn't fair to lose a mutual reality that once sustained the closeness that dementia is now stealing away. It isn't fair to be left alone. It doesn't feel good, and it doesn't bring out the good in us.

The effect of loneliness on physical and emotional health is well established.* The effect on cognitive health, however, has only recently come to light. Loneliness shortens attention span and interferes with judgment and self-control, the very attributes required to deal with a patient's fixations and delusions. Self-control, in fact, is already a limited resource precisely because it requires the same kind of energy involved in any effortful activity, be it emotional, cognitive, or physical, which is why there's so little of it to go around. The same energy needed to resist a pastry or a cigarette is also called on when dealing with someone's delusions and unreasonable demands.

Although caregivers do their best to restrain themselves by applying the "mental brakes" found in the right ventrolateral prefrontal cortex (rVLPFC), it turns out that Alzheimer's not only weakens the patient's rVLPFC, it also impairs the caregiver's ability to exercise self-control. It's unfortunate

---

* Loneliness raises the odds of depression and anxiety. It tampers with the immune system and may be as detrimental to bodily health as obesity, lack of exercise, and high blood pressure. One well-known study suggests that loneliness imposes a physical cost similar to that of smoking fifteen cigarettes a day.

that the very symptoms that add to caregivers' loneliness are those that actually impede them from effectively applying those mental brakes.

Dementia disorders thus constitute a physiological ensnarement that requires caregivers to constantly override their natural impulses and intuitions, even as it robs them of the energy to do so. This leaves many caregivers in what social psychologists call a state of ego depletion. That is to say, they experience their own version of "sundowning." After a long day of regulating patients' emotions, of submitting to the existential and mundane forms of unfairness the disease creates—and in many cases doing all this alone—a caregiver's own cognitive and moral reserves are depleted.

Indeed, as the day goes on, caregivers may increasingly begin to mirror the people they're caring for, though most aren't aware of it. They simply lose control and, afterward, suffer pangs of remorse—which is when they tell themselves to get a grip, to work harder, to be nicer. All understandable sentiments, but they stem from one of our most powerful illusions: the conviction that we have a choice in how we respond.

IN THE PREVIOUS CHAPTER WE saw that people are biologically inclined to believe they possess free will, mainly because consciousness comes with the inexorable conviction that it's in charge of the mind's and body's actions, but it may not be that simple. To adjust our expectations, Patricia Churchland argues that we should rid ourselves of this "absolutist" approach and start thinking about free will in terms of degrees—that is, optimal ranges of decision-making. Evidently, the mind is open to a larger variety of responses at some times than it is at other times.

An example she offers is the relationship between willpower and overeating. Not too long ago, it was assumed that obesity was a question of will, that self-control was all we needed. But this is hardly the whole story. A protein called leptin is known to affect hunger and satiety. Mutations in the leptin gene were first seen to cause overeating in mice, and more recent studies with human participants revealed that leptin, as well as certain genetic predispositions, make people more vulnerable to obesity. Indeed, many situations that we associate with willpower are influenced by biological and environmental factors beyond our control. Willpower isn't something we have or don't have; it's more like an accordion that expands and contracts depending on circumstance.

Precisely because caregiving drains us of energy, I encourage caregivers to get away once in a while—to refuel, to find meaning and pleasure in life. But, as I have learned, not all caregivers jump at the opportunity to take a break from their duties, or feel good when they do. Although I urged Cathy to spend more time at work or with friends, she did so with a certain ambivalence. Yes, it felt good to get away, she said, but she also felt guilty. Why should she enjoy herself when her husband was ill? Wasn't she being selfish and self-indulgent for leaving him alone or in the care of an aide?

Sometimes the hardest part of listening to caregivers is knowing I can't assuage their guilt. When I tell them that they deserve time off, that it will make them better caregivers, many just nod politely. And even when they take my advice and arrange to get away, their guilt rarely dissipates.

Nor can I talk them out of it. I do what I can, but while I tug at reason, guilt tugs at intuition. Many caregivers remain convinced that they're capable of doing what needs to be done without the "crutch" of self-care. They believe they can will themselves to tamp down the anger. They think, "If only I cared enough, were kind enough, were disciplined enough, I could handle this." Regrettably, this self-criticism focuses on what they see as a character flaw. How much more forgiving we would be if we recognized the true source of the problem: the inherent physiological limitations of self-control.

7

My Dinner with Stefan Zweig

Why We Take Patients' Words and Actions Personally

One by one, three French citizens, a man and two women, escorted by a valet with the detached look of a DMV worker, are brought to a room decorated in Second Empire style. They know they have died but not why they've been thrown together. Soon it becomes apparent that they do not get along, and after they confess their crimes they prey on one another's insecurities and weaknesses. The man, whose name is Garcin, is miserable. One woman likes him, the other doesn't. Naturally, he wants the approval of the one who is dismissive. But the more he explains himself, the more she humiliates him. He desperately wants to leave. He rings for the valet, but he doesn't come. Then, without much hope, he approaches the door. He pulls on the knob, and unexpectedly the door opens. Suddenly he's free to go, to leave behind the squabbling and the recriminations. But he hesitates. Finally he gets it. He realizes this is hell and it has nothing to do with torture chambers or fire and brimstone. Hell is other people.

HENRY AND IDA FRANKEL LIVE in a cozy three-bedroom apartment in Manhattan's Washington Heights. Henry, a soft-spoken retired architect of eighty-five, is a short, handsome man with a bald head and small ears. Ida is even shorter, with fine white hair coiled in a bun. Although she is usually smartly turned out, smelling of powder and lavender, only Henry knows how much effort this entails. Whenever he tries to cut her nails, give her a bath, or change her clothes, Ida's small face contorts into something unrecognizable; she becomes like a fierce, cornered animal.

Henry's and Ida's families immigrated to New York from Austria in the 1930s, when both were teenagers. They met at the City College of New York, and in 1953, one year to the day after graduation, they were married. Allowing for the usual ups and downs, their marriage was a good one. They liked the same novels and films and shared a love of chamber music. Their apartment is lined with books and a large collection of Deutsche Grammophon LPs. There isn't a CD in the house because, as Henry explained, they couldn't bear to betray their beloved albums.

While Henry took to American culture right away, Ida continued to miss the Viennese world she had known as a child. And while Henry joined a midlevel architectural firm and embarked on a career, Ida struggled to find her identity. She wanted to be a writer, then a photographer, then a decorator. She wanted, she said, to carve out something of her own, but nothing ever came of it.

In her midseventies, Ida began showing signs of Alzheimer's. Her decline was gradual. She experienced the usual memory loss and attendant confusion, but life went on pretty much as before. Then one day, Henry came home to find Ida speaking to a framed photograph on the mantelpiece. They had many photographs of departed friends and family around the apartment, and Ida began to go from one to another, telling aunts and cousins whatever she happened to be thinking about. After the initial shock wore off, Henry became used to her chatter and resigned himself to this new quirk of hers. He'd obviously known her friends and relatives, and he didn't mind their playing a role in her imaginative life.

Once Ida turned eighty, she also began having conversations with books. Not in the sense of communing with the characters, but with the authors themselves, or, more accurately, with their jacket photos. This Henry could not get used to. He never knew when he might come across Ida sitting across from a book propped upright on the coffee table, speaking to the author photo.

"Thank God," he said, "they didn't speak back to her."

To Proust, she might talk about her childhood in Vienna; to Virginia Woolf, she spoke of her honeymoon and how Henry had once gotten lost in Venice. To Rilke, she spoke about fashion, porcelain, and popular music. Henry never knew what she might say; he just knew that after a while *he* had stopped figuring in her conversations entirely. As time passed, he began to feel like an intruder in his own home. Indeed, aside from occasional comments about shopping and schedules, she barely spoke to him at all, keeping the warmest part of herself for her two-dimensional friends.

By the time Henry and I met, on a cold spring day, he could no longer separate his grief from his consternation. But because of his gentle manner and natural reserve, one could miss the anger simmering beneath his words, an anger directed mostly against himself. Had he been a better husband, he told me toward the end of our first conversation, he might have saved Ida from the bleakness and indignity of Alzheimer's.

"She'll talk to *them* with the tenderness that's missing when she talks to me," a bereft Henry told me.

What do you say to someone whose wife prefers photographs of deceased authors to him?

One morning, Henry awoke to find Ida chattering to Thomas Mann and was struck by the thought that their shared appreciation of certain writers, which had once united them, now put a wedge between them. How was he supposed to compete with the author of *Buddenbrooks*? He couldn't help it: He became envious of the photographs and sometimes eavesdropped. Then, when she accused him of spying, he felt terrible.

Despite how alienating he found his wife's delusions, he remained protective. In fact, he bristled when her doctor or friends suggested medication. As long as she was happy, Henry reasoned, there was no reason to deprive her of a rich inner life.

"At least one of us has a social life," he joked to me.

One sunny afternoon when Henry and I met at the Clois-
ters, he informed me that the night before, Ida had invited a
guest for dinner: the Austrian writer Stefan Zweig, who died
in 1942. "I guess I should feel like a big shot having Stefan
Zweig for dinner," Henry muttered. He didn't bother trying to
sound amused.

The dinner had not gone well. After putting food on the
table, Ida had directed all her remarks to the cover of *The
World of Yesterday* except when she asked Henry to pass a roll
to their guest. This request cracked his self-resolve. "You
have ridiculous delusions!" he shouted. "It's a picture! Pictures do not eat! Your craziness is making me crazy."

Unperturbed, Ida prepared a plate for her guest. But
when she urged Zweig to take a bite, Henry blurted, "I told
you! You can't feed pictures. This is why you need to listen
to me."

Recounting this to me, Henry smiled. "You know, it felt
good telling her."

But the feeling had been quickly replaced by guilt. Ida
sulked and stopped eating. Touched by her vulnerability and
the absurdity of his small victory, Henry had apologized and
begged for forgiveness.

His outburst, he confessed, had left him rattled and miserable. Perplexed by his own behavior, he said, "People talk
about my wife like she has a problem. But it's me. I'm the one
with the problem."

Henry couldn't shake off the sting of Ida's daily rejec-
tions. He knew they weren't personal, but they felt personal.
This was his wife, his friend of more than sixty years. When
he was away from her, he still missed her: her voice, her

scent, her mannerisms. Most of all, he missed feeling useful. Now, when he cooked dinner or helped her dress, she didn't seem to care.

Mocking himself, he told me, "What do I expect? For her to say, 'Ooh, you are such a good husband'?"

Henry was, as he readily admitted, a people pleaser. First he had tried to please a difficult mother and then difficult clients and then, of course, his occasionally disappointed wife. After Ida fell ill, after she no longer even recognized him except as someone who looked after her, he still wanted to make her happy. But he also wanted her to know that he was trying to help. He considered this a weakness, wanting the good opinion of others in order to have a good opinion of himself. And he felt ashamed of trying to win her approval, knowing that his first concern should be her welfare rather than his self-esteem.

HELL MAY BE OTHER PEOPLE in Jean-Paul Sartre's *No Exit*, but tellingly, the unhappy protagonist, Garcin, *chooses* hell; he chooses to be with other people. As long as one of the women thinks badly of him, he cannot leave. Sartre means for us to disapprove of Garcin because he allows other people to define him, thereby forfeiting his chance at authenticity. At first glance, readers might agree with Sartre's assessment. Why should strangers exert such influence over us? Although we accept that we're partially shaped by those around us, we also firmly believe that each of us is capable of self-determination, that a part of us is immune from external influences and is uniquely "us."

This is why we berate ourselves for taking things personally, for wanting the approval of people, even those who are neither cognitively nor emotionally equipped to give it. Sartre would certainly approve of this self-criticism. But as it turns out, the notion that there is a part of ourselves that is entirely separate from others is most likely a fiction.

It's simply not how the brain appears to be designed. The medial prefrontal cortex (MPFC), the part of the brain that is activated when we think about who we are, is also activated when we reflect on how others perceive us. Neurologically speaking, there is no special place in the brain that is hermetically sealed from the influence of other people. Quite the contrary: The self is porous.

Not only is the brain susceptible to outside influences, as Matthew Lieberman has demonstrated, but the region in the brain where identity originates acts as "a superhighway where others influence our lives." Lieberman, in fact, regards the self as "evolution's sneakiest ploy . . . a secret agent" designed to make us receptive to other minds by accommodating their thoughts and ideas. But what makes the self truly sneaky is that it believes an essential part of itself is impervious to outside influences, whereas, in fact, it all too often collapses under the weight of social pressure. This happens not just because we feel a need to belong to a community, but also because evolution has made us into social beings whose brains naturally absorb the worldview of other brains.

Sartre might simply shrug upon learning that the MPFC is the bad actor denying us authenticity. So what if this region of the brain is or isn't activated? What does it matter that we're influenced by external factors? Perhaps this only makes our decisions *more* important, since the tendency to be affected by others can lead us astray. Perhaps we should focus harder on defining ourselves. He might even posit that we can still be "authentic" individuals as long as we choose to be.

But actually we do not *choose* to be preoccupied with other people. The activity of the MPFC is a neural habit. We don't turn on the MPFC when choosing to think about others; we think about others because the MPFC is our brain's default mode.

In other words, social reasoning is as natural as, well, thinking. Evolution could have pushed us toward becoming expert abstract thinkers and problem solvers, but it didn't. Instead, it enhanced our social reasoning in order to help us survive in increasingly complex social networks. It's why we're so preoccupied with one another.

So when caregivers are yelled at, lied to, ignored, unfairly accused, or not recognized, how can this not affect their sense of self? But like Garcin, they choose to remain, and like Garcin, they find themselves consigned to a hell in an ordinary setting, surrounded by familiar objects. Most caregivers, after all, are "tortured" in living rooms and kitchens, rooms that hold memories and trigger old patterns of behavior, rooms that damn them to choose an unhappy or unnerving dynamic over no dynamic at all.

LET'S CONSIDER ANOTHER SCENARIO IN which three people find themselves in a nondescript room, one less ornate than Sartre's. They happen to be volunteers in an experiment, but they have no idea what it entails. So they sit around, waiting. Suddenly one of them spies a ball in a corner. He picks it up and casually tosses it to another person, who then tosses it to the third. Soon they're playing a nice, unhurried game of catch—until, without warning, two of the players decide to stop playing with the third. For no apparent reason, they ignore him, tossing the ball only to each other. The person left out can only watch helplessly as the game continues without him.

As it happens, this interaction *is* the experiment. Two of the people are confederates; the third isn't in on the secret. The game, created by the psychologist Kip Williams, is called Cyberball, and because the stakes are fairly low, we might, picturing ourselves in the role of the third person, believe we would take our exclusion from this silly game in stride. But we would be deluding ourselves if we thought we wouldn't feel unnerved by being left out.

This point was reinforced by Matthew Lieberman, who replicated the Cyberball experiment using functional magnetic resonance imaging (fMRI). He asked people to play *digital* Cyberball with two other players. Although the subjects believed they were playing with real people, they were actually playing with programmed avatars that eventually began to exclude the subject. As expected, a good many of the participants expressed hurt and anger over the rejection. Moreover, brain scans revealed that their dorsal anterior cingulate cortex (dACC), the area in the brain sensitive to social pain, had been activated.

All this could have been predicted. The real surprise came when participants were informed that their "opponents" was a computer programmed to reject them. Even after they knew it was a machine, they still experienced social pain.

I thought about this experiment when Henry confessed that he was jealous of Stefan Zweig. "Jealous of Stefan Zweig!" he repeated incredulously. "Jealous of Stefan Zweig!" He couldn't believe it. But I could. If we can become upset by a computer's rejection, how can we not feel social pain when ignored, dismissed, or accused by people we know and love?

Ida's dementia made her no less a person to Henry, nor did it matter that her other "relationships" were imaginary. What mattered was that Ida was living her life without him. Our biological makeup is so intent on maintaining social connections that the source of the rejection is less important than we might imagine. Biology, after all, is interested not in nuanced thinking but in survival.

Perhaps this is why human beings, along with other mammals, have evolved to feel isolation as painful. Rejection literally hurts. Physical pain and emotional pain might feel different, but they derive from a common neurobiological source. The same dorsal anterior cingulate cortex (dACC) that registers feelings of exclusion also registers physical pain.

If social pain and physical pain are not so distinct in the brain, then perhaps Tylenol can help mend a broken heart. This isn't a glib suggestion. Social psychologists have determined that people who take painkillers instead of placebos (over the course of a few weeks) experience significantly less pain from rejection and isolation. In one experiment, researchers instructed two groups to play Cyberball, with one group taking painkillers and the other group placebos.

Not only did participants taking painkillers report lower levels of agitation from rejection, but brain scans also revealed significantly less activity in their dACC.

The neuroscientist Jaak Panksepp, who coined the term "affective neuroscience," convincingly argues that our attachment system piggybacks on our physical pain system by using the body's natural opioid secretions. This seems like a sensible plan, given that isolation or separation from a group threatens survival. Social pain is clearly an evolutionary tool, an adaptive signal that urges us to keep close, the better to improve our chances of survival. Just as physical pain alerts us to something that may be harmful, social pain alerts us to the danger of isolation.

Again, this makes evolutionary sense because without the pain of separation and isolation, a baby wouldn't bother to cry out and a mother wouldn't know her child was in trouble. Analogously, if the mother's dACC is damaged, she is far less likely to respond to her child's cries. In fact, in one unpleasant experiment, rats with lesions in the dACC seemed indifferent to caring for their offspring, and only 20 percent of the babies survived.

Because providing care and receiving care are biologically linked, Ida's rejection of Henry's overtures naturally made him feel uncared for. But he could not disengage. In fact, he only tried harder to reestablish their connection. So while Sartre believed that the self can be authentic only when it is untethered to other selves, biology has other plans. Indeed, there is a reason for the neural similarity between thinking about oneself and thinking about others. It allows us, as the neuropsychologist Nicholas Humphrey says, to hone and practice our social reasoning skills, not as a means to "know thyself" but to become better at knowing and understanding others.

Of course, one of the cruelties of Alzheimer's is that caregivers' adaptive instincts now work against them. So when Henry feels hurt by Ida's loss of interest in him, his pain no longer serves its natural purpose of connecting him to his wife. As Henry ruefully observed to me during one of our last meetings: "I suppose I should be happy that she's happy. She has her books and her pictures, and when I play music for her, she's in heaven. She really doesn't need anything else."

He then fell silent for a moment. "But how do I get used to the fact that she has no use for me?"

8

The Mastermind

Why We Continue to Rely on Reason

IN *DESCARTES' ERROR*, THE NEUROSCIENTIST ANTONIO DAMASIO introduces us to an unusual patient. Elliot is a businessman in his midthirties. His memory, computational skills, and geographic orientation are all excellent. There is nothing wrong with his learning ability or logic and language skills. He knows right from wrong and is personable, considerate, and quietly humorous. He also happens to be up to date on politics, current affairs, and the economy. All the cognitive tests agree: There is nothing wrong with Elliot. And yet Elliot's life is falling apart.

Some years earlier a benign tumor had appeared in the front part of Elliot's brain. Surgeons removed the tumor, as well as the affected frontal lobe tissue. Elliot suffered no ill effects physically, but gradually he began to lose interest in his work. He became unable to manage his time, starting new projects but unable to finish them. Eventually he lost his job. He then struck out on his own, starting new business ventures, sometimes with disreputable partners. He lost his savings and then his wife. He married again and divorced again. He drifted and couldn't find work. He became a man who could no longer make reasonable decisions in either business or social situations.

Damasio was stumped. Why was a man who performed well on every cognitive test incapable of functioning in the real world? After a time, Damasio began to wonder if he might be looking at the problem from the wrong angle. Thinking over how Elliot talked about his failed marriages, his stalled career, and the loss of his friends, Damasio was struck by the fact that he always did so without regret or annoyance. Although puzzled by what had happened to him, Elliot seemed neither anxious nor upset. Was it possible that he was putting all his energy into controlling his inner emotional turmoil? Or was there simply no turmoil to begin with? Damasio didn't know. What he did know is that *he* was more upset about Elliot's life than Elliot was, and this caused him to doubt Elliot's emotional capacity.

Spurred by this thought, Damasio decided to try something new. He presented Elliot with distressing visual stimuli: a house burning and people injured in horrible accidents, images that ordinarily elicit strong emotional reactions. Elliot, however, showed no discomfort. Intellectually he knew the pictures depicted terror and suffering, but physiologically (and therefore emotionally), he registered no distress. His breathing, heart rate, and brain waves were essentially unaffected. Then, using brain imaging techniques, Damasio confirmed that Elliot had no emotional stake in what was happening to him or around him. The problem, Damasio concluded, was that Elliot was able "to know but not to feel."

Although I had never run across anyone like Elliot, I couldn't help thinking about him when I heard about someone who seemed to be his exact counterpart. She was an elderly Chinese woman with Alzheimer's disease. Her name was Min, and her granddaughter, whom I'll call Julia, had come to my office one day to discuss their relationship. In the light streaming through the window, I noticed the touching contrast between Julia's round, adolescent-looking features and the familiar harried expression, that of a much older caregiver.

Julia, I soon learned, was sleeping in two-hour shifts, a pattern that began after she moved out of Min's apartment and arranged for twenty-four-hour care. She couldn't sleep because she knew that her phone might ring at any moment. Min would call either to demand to know why Julia wasn't there or to complain about the incompetent aides who apparently did nothing but wear out the rugs. One, Min declared, was dumb as a goat; another, useless as a cow; another, lazy as a pig.

The aides also phoned at all hours, upset by Min's constant abuse. Knowing how woefully underpaid these women were, Julia felt responsible for their misery, believing that Min's anger was meant for her because she had left. But the calls Julia dreaded most were from the supervisor of the Chinese healthcare agency in Queens. Every few weeks, the supervisor warned Julia that her grandmother's punitive behavior toward the aides had to stop. Six or seven had already quit, and soon there would be no one left to send over. In short, her grandmother had to stop acting "crazy," or else.

At this point, Julia paused and gave me an exasperated look. "How can I instruct my grandmother about anything? She has Alzheimer's!"

"The supervisor doesn't get it?" I asked.

Julia shrugged. "You'd think so, but it's not that simple."

Alzheimer's, Julia explained, was a cultural blind spot in the Chinese community. In fact, in Chinese the term for dementia is *chi dai zheng,* which translates to "crazy and catatonic" or "insane and idiotic." For her grandmother's generation, neurological disorders did not really exist. Bad behavior was simply bad behavior. The person, not the brain, was responsible.

To people who knew Min, she was still her old irascible self. Alzheimer's may have made buying food, paying rent, and attending to her mail more difficult, but that didn't mean something was wrong. Nonetheless, Min sensed that she was not quite herself. Worried that people might think less of her, she resorted to excessive vigilance. Everyone, she warned Julia, was after something, even those who wanted to help her. Her friends, her neighbors, her nephew, all were suspect.

"She's worse than ever," Julia told me. "I don't know what to do."

I nodded, thinking: If the supervisor of the healthcare agency couldn't see that Min was suffering from a disease, how could Julia expect others to see it?

As if following my thoughts, Julia blurted out: "Everyone sees her mood swings as Min not getting her own way. Even her paranoia seems normal. She always distrusted people, always took offense. People just think Min is being Min."

MIN HAD GROWN UP IN a village outside Shenzhen and arrived in the United States in her late thirties. Determined not to seem like an ignorant, unworldly immigrant, she tamped down her insecurity and adopted the persona of someone in the know. For forty years she had shown to the world a tough, unyielding, confident face. Once she formed an opinion, it was intractable. She didn't care that people thought she wasn't nice. Niceness was an American preoccupation; it left you vulnerable, and vulnerability was a luxury Min could not afford.

Alzheimer's only reinforced Min's disposition. Even Julia could not be sure where her grandma's habitual defenses ended and her dementia began—because on some level the distinction didn't exist. As Julia quietly admitted to me, the person she spent the most time convincing about her grandmother's illness was herself.

I told her that I had heard the same comment from other caregivers and obligingly asked what she meant.

She laughed. "I'm still trying to figure that one out."

Partly it had to do with Min's memory, which had always been something of a mystery to Julia. When she was little, she had to tread carefully because Min interpreted every frown or gesture of impatience as willful disobedience and immediately became enraged. On occasion, she even hit her with a hairbrush or whatever object was handy. Corporal punishment was not unusual in Min's day, and Julia always forgave these outbursts.

In truth, what bothered her more than the hitting and yelling was their apparent erasure. The next morning, Min would never allude to what she'd done; she'd simply slide a plate of food over to her as if to say, "Let's move on." And because such eruptions were not acknowledged, Julia never felt entirely safe.

Now that Alzheimer's had a grip on Min, the pattern continued. Min would lose her temper and scream, but fifteen minutes later she'd offer Julia a piece of fruit or a cup of tea. Had the incident been forgotten? Julia couldn't be sure. Was Min once again avoiding an unpleasant situation of her own making? Or was Alzheimer's causing her to forget? If Min could not remember, how could Julia be sure she was doing the right thing? How could she know if she made her grandma happy?

Listening to this young woman torture herself, I asked why she was bearing all the responsibility alone. Julia thought for a moment and then plunged into her complicated family history. Min, it turns out, was not her real grandmother. Julia's mother had had an affair with a man who already had a wife and family. He had spent little time with Julia or her mother, who was cold and indifferent to her inconvenient child. So Julia had ended up in the care of the permanent babysitter her father had hired: Min.

Having never felt unconditional love from either of her parents, Julia took nothing for granted and sought to prove herself to everyone, especially the woman she had come to regard as her grandmother. And Min, who had no family of her own except for nieces and nephews, returned Julia's love. But for Min, love meant there could be no boundaries between them.

By the time Julia came to see me, she felt pulled in all directions. Not only did she have to deal with aides threatening to quit, not only was the agency supervisor threatening to remove them, she also had to repeatedly assure Min that she had not been abandoned.

"I guess this isn't how a twentysomething is supposed to live," Julia noted.

"True," I said, adding, "Your grandmother is lucky to have you."

"I am the one who is lucky," Julia said earnestly. "She saved me. Without her I don't know who or where I would be."

When I heard this, I worried about all the ways her gratitude could be exploited by the disease, and I ended our first meeting with a gentle insistence that Julia come back whenever she felt overwhelmed.

I can't say I was surprised when I heard from her in less than a week. Her favorite aide, the one she relied on the most, had abruptly announced that she was leaving, and Julia was in a panic. This aide (I'll call her Yu Yan), unlike previous aides, had actually made an attempt to understand the disease. She acknowledged that Min had a problem "with her brain" and sometimes affectionately impersonated her to make Julia laugh.

Which is why it jarred Julia to learn that Yu Yan was ready to quit. She rushed over to Min's apartment to find the aide in tears. She was crying not because Min had yelled or tried to throw her out, but because she had told Yu Yan that she could not be trusted. Min accused Yu Yan of staying only because she had a sick child at home and could not afford to lose her job.

"The problem with your grandma," Yu Yan told Julia between sobs, "is not that she's mean or has a disease. The real problem is that she is still very reasonable."

The observation shook Julia. She realized that no matter how crazy her grandmother acted, Julia still believed there was a logic to her behavior, a weird, misshapen logic perhaps, but one with an undercurrent of sense. Telling me this, Julia gave me a sly smile and said: "My grandma is more than reasonable. She is a mastermind."

Seeing my amused expression, she continued: "Listen to what my grandma can do."

Evidently it wasn't the first time that Min had used personal information to get her way. A previous aide had been told to take the weekend off because Julia was coming to stay over. It wasn't true, but when the aide wanted to confirm with Julia, Min had snapped, "What, because I am old, you don't trust me? I don't want to deal with people who don't trust me." The aide, young and inexperienced, wavered. And Min knew just the right thing to say to cinch the deal: "Why would you want to spend the weekend with me when you have two young children at home?"

"I'm so tired of it all," Julia confided.

"Of course you are," I said. "It can't be easy being manipulated all these years."

Surprised, Julia asked, "How can my grandma be manipulative when she has Alzheimer's? Does the word even apply?"

"It's not that simple," I said. "Just because Min has Alzheimer's doesn't mean that she can't scheme." Julia looked dubious.

Many caregivers have given me the same look. Most people think that Alzheimer's impairs reason because it interferes with cognition and executive functions. It certainly does that, but this doesn't mean that victims become helpless. They remain capable of getting their own way, of making us believe them, of sucking us into arguments. Nonetheless, we continue to underestimate patients because of our own understanding of what reason entails.

WHEN DAMASIO FIRST EXAMINED ELLIOT, he did not immediately grasp Elliot's problem. Like all of us, as he admits, he was inclined to see reason as something separate from our gangly, unruly emotions. This, of course, has been the received wisdom from Plato's time to the twenty-first century. Emotions may give life color and even make life worth living, but when it comes to decision-making, we believe they interfere with reasoning. This is why Elliot's doctors could not diagnose him. How could someone so composed, with cognitive faculties in full working order, behave so irrationally? It defied common sense.

Damasio's insight, now backed by decades of research,

proves that there is no such thing as "pure" reason. Reason and emotion, far from being distinct, actually overlap. Yet for the longest time, scientists thought that the neocortex, which deals with "higher" processes (willpower, nuanced thinking, high-level decision-making), worked separately from the subcortex, where our "low" processes (biological regulation and emotion) are found. Naturally it was also assumed that when big problems came up, the neocortex did all the heavy lifting while the components of our more basic nature took a back seat. As Damasio put it, we seem to have an "upstairs/downstairs" narrative of the brain. But, in fact, this story does not match the neural reality: The "low" or "downstairs" compartments are just as essential as the neocortex for rational decision-making.

Today we know the mind and body are not physiologically divisible. The mind, whatever else it is, is an amalgam of the brain, the body, and the environment in which they all coexist. For Damasio, "the cortical networks on which feelings rely include not only the traditionally acknowledged collection of brain structures known as the limbic system but also some of the brain's prefrontal cortices, and, most importantly, the brain sectors that map and integrate signals from the body."

These signals, which constitute the body's physiological response to experience, inform us whether something is good or bad, safe or threatening. Damasio calls these responses—e.g., a rapid heartbeat when feeling anxious—"somatic markers," and he argues that they are indispensable to decision-making. Indeed, the more we learn about the brain, the more evident it becomes that emotions necessarily factor into how we think. Without preferences and feelings, our mind would have to sift through numerous options, one seeming no better than another.

In Elliot's case, the neural connection between cognition and emotion had somehow been severed. Elliot could reason, but his decisions had no real-life application. Just as Funes's perfect memory left him unable to carve out meaning from his experiences, Elliot's inability to respond emotionally to an experience left him unable to assign value to it. He couldn't finish or commit to anything because no one task or person was more important than another.

Although Min would have failed the cognitive tests that Elliot had sailed through, she often performed better in life precisely because, unlike Elliot, she could *feel* her way through a situation. Having somatic markers to guide her, she was no one's fool. If anything, she was the one doing the fooling, relying on emotional strategies that had served her in the past.

If too much emotion made Min suspicious of people, the absence of emotion made Elliot trust people who wouldn't think twice about betraying him. In neither case, however, were their respective modes of irrational behavior viewed as neurological problems. Because Elliot seemed intelligent and "with it," his behavior made people think he was indifferent, lazy, and wrong-headed. Min, on the other hand, was seen as mean, obstreperous, and impetuous, since her decisiveness and determination did not appear to derive from a mind that was slowing down.

WHEN JULIA HAD RUSHED HOME after Min tricked the aide into leaving, they fought. Didn't Min realize she was costing Julia time and energy? Hadn't Julia told her time and again how hard it was to get help? Didn't Min know how long it had been since Julia went out and did something for herself? Min refused to listen. She was the one who had been wronged. She was the one who had been abandoned by an ungrateful granddaughter, a person too selfish to spend the day with her grandmother.

At which point, Julia stalked out, leaving her grandma alone.

Telling me this, Julia was contrite. She regretted her outburst, her indignation, and the fact that she had temporarily abandoned her grandmother. What she had to do, she said earnestly, was learn to let go of her emotions.

Although Julia believed that emotions were clouding her judgment, I believed that her anger that day was an adaptive warning that she was reaching the end of her rope. It was the culmination of a lifetime of incidents in which she felt controlled by her grandma, incidents about which she had kept silent. When she walked out on Min, she was choosing her own welfare over her grandma's needs, and, far from interfering with reason, anger finally helped her set a boundary. Anger, I reassured her, did not make her a bad person; it was a healthy response to an unhealthy situation.

Because Min's somatic markers remained intact, so did her sense of right and wrong. When she felt opposed, mistreated, or condescended to, her emotional antennae quivered and she responded in both forceful and nuanced ways. This emotional awareness, exacerbated by Alzheimer's, prevented Julia from seeing Min as a person impaired by disease. And when they argued, Julia's own somatic markers made her feel that she was still in the presence of the formidable woman whom she needed to please, to whom she had to prove herself worthy of trust and love.

Healthcare professionals often joke that they have never won an argument with an Alzheimer's patient. The implication, of course, is that such arguments are futile because patients cannot follow our logic. But what people often fail to mention is that arguing is also inevitable. We argue with our patients not because we cannot accept their limitations, but because we're both provoked and encouraged by their strengths. Patients can be quite nimble at defending themselves, serving up one rebuttal after another even after they've lost the thread of an argument. Because emotions carry them along.

Paul Slovic, a researcher who studies bias and decision-making, explains that all of us are partial to taking emotional shortcuts when making decisions. The question "What do I think?" is implicitly replaced in our mind with "How do I feel?" This is called the *affect heuristic*. With a nod toward Damasio, Slovic suggests that our emotional evaluations and physical states are intertwined and that both are key indicators of decision-making. Since we're all inclined to lead with our feelings, we tend to see the emotional behavior of dementia patients as normal, especially when they argue with us, since they, like us, still lead with their emotions. And because these heuristics don't go away when dementia surfaces (if anything, they become more useful), the emotional thread of their arguments doesn't necessarily change.

In fact, Alzheimer's can sometimes make patients seem even more formidable. Min, unencumbered by context and logic, had something enviable: certainty. And this feeling of certainty, which is both a personality trait and a product of Alzheimer's, propelled her through arguments. She either immediately forgot inconvenient facts or she wasn't able to process them, and thus her unreasonable demands appeared to issue from a powerful, if bullheaded, woman rather than from a victim of a brain disorder.

So if pure reason does not exist and emotions are an essential part of reasoning, how can we distinguish between the faulty reasoning of a healthy brain and the impaired reasoning of a damaged one? It's no wonder Julia sometimes half-jokingly questioned the very existence of her grandma's Alzheimer's.

Julia was desperate. She didn't want to comply every time her grandmother called, but she also didn't want to live with Min's anger because whenever Min accused her of not visiting or of not being on her side, Julia's lifelong fear of disappointing her invariably surfaced. She then felt compelled to plead her case, insisting that she often visited. Min, however, took this insistence as an argument, and arguments were only more proof of Julia's disobedience and betrayal.

What could she do? I told Julia what I usually tell other caregivers: A little fibbing can go a long way. She could promise to visit and not follow through. But Julia felt it was wrong to lie, and she was convinced she would get caught. "If it's important to her, she'll remember," she said.

I explained that what was paramount for Min was less

the truth than the feeling of being wanted. To stop her grand-mother from getting angry meant learning to address the emotions beneath the accusations. Julia had to learn to "speak Alzheimer's," which clinically means focusing on a patient's feelings rather than on the facts, which for the patient change from moment to moment.

Although Julia grasped what I was saying, she couldn't quite accept it. The idea of forsaking the truth when dealing with a loved one is not something that comes easily. I was at a loss. How could I get Julia to shake off her feelings of inad-equacy and guilt when she believed everything her grand-mother said?

I was still worrying about this when Julia invited me to visit her and Min on the Chinese New Year. I gladly accepted the invitation, hoping that it would present an opportunity to demonstrate that Min's convictions were as mercurial as her moods.

ON THE APPOINTED DAY, I dressed in red (considered a lucky color in China) and brought along a large coffee cake, oranges, and dumplings, which are also associated with good fortune. I had no idea how Min would receive me as I ner-vously rode the subway to Queens. Perhaps she'd see me as another intruder, and I would just make things worse for Julia. Happily, she greeted me with a big hug and dug right into the basket of food. "This is too much," she said, clearly pleased, and insisted that we immediately eat the coffee cake. She made a pot of tea and handed me a small red envelope with money inside, which is traditionally given on the Chinese New Year. She seemed delighted when I gratefully accepted the envelope.

Min was small, frail, but she was still agile. If Damasio had been disarmed by Elliot's composure, I was taken with how emotionally attuned Min seemed. She was amused when I was amused and eagerly nudged Julia to explain whatever struck my curiosity. As a host, she radiated warmth, her eyes glowing with purpose. The fact that we didn't speak the same language did not deter us. Even when Julia took a break from translating, Min and I gesticulated wildly and seemed to understand each other. She was like any grandmother, wanting to feed her guests and eager to brag about her grandchildren.

During all this hubbub, Julia looked apologetic and uncomfortable, but I assured her that I was used to being manhandled by small, elderly immigrants—in my case, Russian Jews. By now I'd been around enough dementia patients to appreciate their ability to shift between confusion and amiability, which sometimes made them appear beguilingly "with it." What I didn't expect, however, was how endearing I'd find Min or how easily she would win me over with her obvious affection for Julia, taking every opportunity to touch, kiss, and caress her. At one point they stood arm in arm, almost melting into each other.

Looking at them, I remarked how happy Julia seemed. "Yes," Julia responded brightly. "She's my little dumpling, my little marshmallow. She has her own smile for me, a 'home smile.'"

As the evening progressed, I became increasingly touched

by Julia's predicament. How could she distance herself from a relationship that was as loving and reassuring as it was unhealthy? Seeing them together, I felt guilty for what I was about to do. Nonetheless, I asked Min how often Julia visited and slept over. Julia gave me a nervous smile but dutifully translated my question.

Min replied, "Almost every day," and reached for Julia's hand. Julia looked shocked.

I then asked Min if anyone else helped her out. Min glanced at Julia and replied, "We help each other."

"But is there anyone else?" I asked.

"No," she said, decisively.

Julia now nudged her grandmother: "What about the aides?"

"Ah," Min said, as though she'd just remembered. "They are very nice."

Julia laughed and asked if she was sure about that. Min shrugged and said that although she didn't need them, they were decent, professional women. Again, Julia looked surprised. She explained to me that this was typical of Min when she was in a good mood. Of course, in a bad mood, she went on to say, Min thought that everyone was lined up against her.

Just as I was thinking to myself how well this little demonstration was going, Julia took Min's hand. They spoke softly for a few seconds. Then Julia, with tears in her eyes, told me what Min had said: "In our next lifetime, I will come and find you. I will always look for you, and we will be together."

I could see that Julia believed that somehow her grandmother understood that Julia was the only person who stood by her. Seeing them together, I was struck by their resemblance. Their features weren't similar, but their faces expressed both melancholy and contentment. Was this the moment to remind Julia to believe only in *this* Min and not in the paranoid Min who might reemerge at any time? The sight of them together told me I could no more successfully convince Julia that she should stop believing her grandmother than Julia could convince her grandmother of how often she visited.

WE EXPECT THE "HEALTHY" MIND to be reasonable when it comes to what we believe and disbelieve. But beliefs are intrinsically tied to feelings, and how we feel is often at the mercy of how others feel. When Min felt good, so did Julia. And when Min said nice things to her, Julia believed her unreservedly. Likewise, when Min felt agitated or paranoid, so did Julia. Sadly, all the harsh things that Min accused her of fed into Julia's conviction that she wasn't doing enough for her grandma.

Julia believed Min because the mind is built to believe— believing, in fact, is automatic. We process and comprehend statements by first assuming them to be true. We do this because it is easier on the brain to accept a statement than to question it, which is why we readily take what people say at face value. And even when caregivers know their loved ones have dementia, even when they know they shouldn't fall for what their spouses or parents or grandparents say, they still cannot help but believe them.

How well I understand such credulity. In the year I spent

with Mr. Kessler, I too, despite knowing better, believed what he told me, even when he promised not to use the stove or leave the house by himself. And if, by the time I met Julia, I had stopped believing in a patient's promises, it wasn't because I had become wise; it was because I was not close to that particular patient. But Julia didn't have that luxury. She was as close to her grandmother as anyone could be.

As I rode the subway home that night, I realized that I, too, yearned for a reality that was at odds with the facts. I wanted Julia not to take Min's accusations to heart. I wanted Julia to look at the situation logically, to face reality in order to be spared any more grief.

But that was presumptuous of me. The Min who showed Julia affection and kindness was no less real than the Min who yelled and derided her. How could I ask Julia to choose which Min to believe? To dismiss one would entail dismissing the other. For Julia, Min was not composed of different parts, some to be trusted more than others. When we engage with people we know and love, we feel the presence of an essential self—not a fractured, intermittently reliable brain.

Believing Min, even if it caused Julia guilt and anguish, might seem an error in judgment, but as I have learned over the years, what can appear unreasonable and self-sabotaging to outsiders can actually constitute a rational trade-off for caregivers. The pain Julia felt because she took Min's hurtful words to heart was still less painful than seeing Min as someone whose words she could now and forever dismiss. How could I, someone who had no history with Min, possibly determine what was or was not reasonable for Julia?

9

Ah Humanity

Why We Attribute Intention to Patients' Behaviors

SOMETIMES CAREGIVERS ASK ME WHAT BOOKS MIGHT HELP them make sense of what they're going through. Generally, they have in mind the various guidebooks that offer practical advice. I'm perfectly happy to recommend such books, as I am a few novels and stories that deal specifically with Alzheimer's and other dementia disorders. But to my mind, it is not literature about dementia disorders that captures the existential strain, the strangeness, and the uncanny yet still ordinary world of the disease. Rather, it's those works of fiction that obliquely approach the problems of existence by slightly heightening and distorting reality that seem to distill the caregiver's experience.

Consider the sad, strange dynamic between what is, in a manner of speaking, a caregiver and a patient in Herman Melville's "Bartleby, the Scrivener." In this story, an elderly Wall Street lawyer, circa 1853, decides to hire an additional scrivener to copy legal documents. He places an advertisement, and one morning finds on his doorstep "a motionless young man . . . pallidly neat, pitiably respectable, incurably forlorn!"

At first, Bartleby is a godsend. Quiet, hardworking, and steady, he copies "by sun-light and by candle-light . . . silently, palely, mechanically." But then, one day, when our narrator asks him to examine a short document, Bartleby replies, "I would prefer not to." The narrator cannot believe his ears. He repeats the request but receives the same response. Because Bartleby betrays no emotion or sign of impertinence, his employer forgives his insubordination. A few days later, he again asks Bartleby to perform a task, and again Bartleby politely declines. "I prefer not to," he says mildly.

Any other man, the narrator assures us, would have been immediately dismissed. "But there was something about Bartleby that not only strangely disarmed me, but in a wonderful manner touched and disconcerted me."

Who is this peculiar man who refuses to entertain reasonable requests from his increasingly perturbed employer? We don't know, because the narrator learns nothing about him except that he has no home. Although Bartleby has now stopped working, he remains in place, staring out the window at a brick wall. The narrator is at a loss. His other clerks are growing resentful, and clients are beginning to wonder. But his pleas make no impression on the man. So he gives Bartleby six days to quit the premises. On the sixth day, however,

Bartleby is still there. Veering between impatience, irritation, and disbelief, the narrator hits upon a desperate solution: Instead of forcibly ejecting Bartleby from his office, he'll relocate his legal practice to another building, thereby leaving the problem of Bartleby behind.

The narrator leaves and Bartleby remains. Some time later, the narrator learns that Bartleby has been evicted but continues to hang around the building. He hurries over to his old office and pleads with Bartleby to leave. He even offers to take Bartleby home with him, but Bartleby prefers not to leave. What does the narrator do? He decides to take a vacation; he simply cannot understand or deal with a man who resolutely prefers not to take care of himself.

ALTHOUGH THE NARRATOR MAY NOT know what to make of Bartleby, there has been no shortage of critics who think they do. For some readers, Bartleby is a stoic victim of capitalism; for others, a rebellious artist victimized by a bourgeois culture; for still others, a Christlike figure sent to redeem his worldly, materialistic employer. Or perhaps he's a symbol of loneliness in an absurd and meaningless universe, whose presence mirrors the isolation in American society?

In our contemporary, diagnosis-ready culture, Bartleby would be assigned a mental or neurological illness. Surely such affectless, passive, noncommunicative behavior signals a schizoid personality disorder or fits somewhere on the autistic spectrum. But isn't this also a way of rendering a mystery more palatable by using terms we're familiar with?

While many readers and critics like to see themselves in

Bartleby, I see myself as the hapless narrator. Nothing quite brings me back to my caregiving days so viscerally as the lawyer's desperate and futile efforts to help the pale scrivener. It is the narrator's desperation that produces their comically one-sided relationship, since Bartleby neither appreciates his concern nor asks for it. The narrator may have position and money, but it's Bartleby who seems in control.

For me, their dynamic is not that of a powerful employer and a vulnerable worker but that of a well-meaning "normal" mind hopelessly trying to make sense of a mind utterly different from its own. The narrator is so sincere, so impassioned, so intent on getting to the bottom of Bartleby's behavior that he doesn't recognize the futility of his *own* behavior. And even when he grasps that his questions will always be met with Bartleby's invincible "I prefer not to," he persists.

Is this any different from how most caregivers behave? Even when we know there's no good answer, we continue to ask our patients: Why don't you listen to me? Why are you hiding the toilet paper? Why are you picking up garbage on the street? Why do you keep wearing the same dirty sweater when I put out a clean one?

Because "Bartleby, the Scrivener" is by turns comical, absurd, and sad, it may feel disturbingly familiar to caregivers. Don't we, as caregivers, vent our anger despite realizing that a loved one has already forgotten the reason we're upset or cannot follow what we're saying? Nonetheless, like Melville's narrator, we also persist. How fitting, then, that Melville's narrator, not unlike the caregiver, is in some ways needier than the person he's trying to help. Even the fact that he's trying to do good makes it hard for him to see how ineffectual he is. He chases after Bartleby not just for answers but also for validation, connection, and ultimately forgiveness.

As for those critics who believe the narrator is inflicting tyrannical social norms on poor Bartleby, they've probably never found themselves in a comparable situation. It's incredibly hard to rescue people from themselves without trying to impose one's own reality on them. Like some dementia patients, Bartleby does not accede but retreats even deeper into his own world, leaving his employer both frustrated and sympathetic. Bartleby, the employer muses, must be terribly lonely; and imagining the depth of such loneliness, he can't help feeling a "fraternal melancholy."

But *is* Bartleby lonely? Who knows? All we know is that the narrator's assumptions reveal more about him than about the scrivener. Most of us, of course, assume the part of the narrator because our mind, like his, is in the deduction business. That is, we are always looking for reasons, motivations, and beliefs in order to make sense of people's behavior.

This deduction business is so serious that it begins very early in our development. Consider what happens when we stick out our tongue at a baby; the baby usually sticks her tongue out at us. Babies do this because our "mirror neurons" literally mirror the behavior of others. If we see someone pick up a cup of coffee, our mirror neurons automatically represent this movement to our brain as if we were picking up the coffee ourselves. The mirroring impulse or "mimicry system" is, in fact, our brain's first step to understanding other people.

We simulate people both with our brain and with our body. We clench when someone experiences a shock and we cringe when others are humiliated. We literally feel other people's pain, because our automatic nervous systems react to their suffering. Our faces, though we may not realize it, are busily copying the reactions of others. (Tellingly, people injected with Botox are not as good at detecting and understanding emotions, precisely because their facial muscles cannot imitate others' expressions.) And if we take a painkiller, which, as we know, helps alleviate social pain, we become less empathetic upon seeing other people's manifestations of rejection or discomfort. And this automatic mirroring, which enables empathy, may actually become problematic for many caregivers.

One caregiver, whom I'll call Shelley, told me she can barely look when her mother tries to read a book or magazine. Her mother, once a brilliant teacher and voracious reader, now seems lost and sad when she turns the pages. "I can't imagine what my mother is feeling," Shelley told me a few times. She really *cannot* imagine it. Nonetheless, she can't help trying to feel what her mother is going through. The instant she perceives her mother's sadness, her mirror neurons not only simulate it, they also cause Shelley to assume they're sharing the same sadness.

She is far from the only one to feel what psychologists call "emotional contagion," which is a by-product of our mimicry system. While empathy seems essential to good caregiving, it can also have, as the psychologist Paul Bloom notes, a surprising drawback. Because egocentricity is "embodied," our understanding of other people begins with ourselves. The pain we automatically feel in response to what we perceive as other people's pain can fool us into thinking that we understand that pain. But the truth is, we don't really know. Shelley may believe that she understood what her mother was feeling, but was she right? Was her mother grieving for herself in the same way that her daughter was? To what degree did she have the capacity to appreciate what she had lost? And how long would it be before she moved on to feeling something else while her daughter was still mired in sadness?

MIRRORING PEOPLE IS ONLY ONE path the brain takes to understand others. Another, somewhat more sophisticated path deploys social reasoning to interpret behavior. Psychologists call this "mind reading," which refers to the tendency to look for intentions, desires, and beliefs when deciphering others. "Mind reading" comes so naturally to us that we have very little control over how or when it's triggered. In the elegant Heider-Simmel triangle experiment, participants were asked to watch shapes moving about at random on a white screen. As it turned out, they didn't observe passively. After a while, they began to see a drama unfold. The randomly moving shapes became distinct characters: bullies, victims, heroes, villains, and the like. Individual shapes began to possess emotions, agendas, and intentions.

Years later, when scientists could perform an MRI of the brain, they replicated the experiment and observed that the mind-reading areas in the medial prefrontal cortex, the dorsomedial prefrontal cortex, the tempoparietal junction, and the posterior cingulate were all activated by the shapes on the screen.

Why are we so "intention-happy," so willing to attribute purpose to randomly moving geometric shapes? The answer involves perhaps our brain's greatest evolutionary aspiration:

prediction. As far as the brain is concerned, there is no more crucial aspect to survival than predicting what other minds are up to and why. And since the only way we can make predictions is to see others as willful rather than mindless, we intuitively attribute purpose to them. For the philosopher Daniel Dennett, this "intentional stance" interprets "behavior as though it were enacted by a rational agent whose actions are the product of choice, deliberation, belief, and above all purpose."

This intuition is so pressing that we talk to, or more often yell at, our phones, cars, computers, though not, perhaps, for the reasons we assume. As long as physical objects continue to function in predictable ways, the brain treats them as inanimate, but as soon as they misfire or fall short of our expectations, the mind-reading areas of the brain are triggered, and suddenly we believe that we're seeing things that exhibit preferences and intentions.

This propensity for "mind reading" is what makes it hard for Melville's narrator not to attribute purpose to Bartleby's singular apathy. As the story unfolds, it's not only Bartleby who spirals downward; it's the narrator as well. Like so many caregivers, he vacillates between thinking that his "patient" suffers from an "innate and incurable disorder" (and thus needs to be indulged) and thinking he's simply a stubborn, perverse figure (and thus needs to be straightened out). Despite feeling that Bartleby means no harm, the narrator is also "strangely goaded" by him. Surely Bartleby knows what he's doing. Even his impressive passivity seems intentional.

This feeling is shared by most caregivers, who, though they might "know" that patients do not act out on purpose, nonetheless feel that they do. How can caregivers *not* feel this way when we, as human beings, attribute motivations to geometric silhouettes? Of course they're going to see intention in surly, capricious patients. It is, in fact, patients' unpredictable behavior (switching between anger and calm, lucidity and confusion) that triggers us to see a willful, determined mind rather than an impaired brain. It's only when patients become consistently passive or docile that caregivers stop seeing intention, which naturally makes it easier to accept the disease.

PROXIMITY, TOO, AFFECTS HOW WE perceive other minds. Movie buffs may remember Orson Welles in *The Third Man* standing on top of a stalled Ferris wheel in Vienna, gazing down on a crowd of tiny figures scurrying about far beneath him ("dots," he calls them), declaiming that they don't matter (so what does it matter if the penicillin he sells them is fake, then?). In fact, the farther we're removed from others, the less likely it is that our brains will engage in "mind reading." That's why it's generally far less distressing for soldiers to kill people remotely by using missiles or drones; they don't see minds, they just see bodies.

Of course, most caregivers have neither the physical nor psychological luxury of distance. Those who do have some distance, such as Lara's husband, Misha, whom we met in chapter 2, end up viewing patients less emotionally. It was because Misha wasn't the one taking care of Mila or burdened by her obsessions that he more easily accepted Alzheimer's. Once he learned that Mila was sick, he saw the disease rather than her histrionics. "If you think about it, it's sad," Misha had told me, with Lara beside him. "For me not to see her as a manipulative person, I had to stop seeing 'Mila' and start seeing a sick brain."

Lara had nodded, but added that for her it was just the opposite. It was hard to stop treating Mila as someone who knew what she was doing. It would have been equivalent to acknowledging that Mila was no longer, as Lara put it, a "person-person." Misha and Lara had in their own way summed up the ethical paradox of caring for people with dementia—namely, the dichotomy the disease forces upon us: personhood versus illness.

It seems cruel that we have to choose, but it's a choice rooted in our biology. Distinct, unconscious processes cause us to see the physical world differently from the mental world. We are, after all, dualistic creatures. We perceive the physical world as abiding by preordained laws (either mechanical or biological), while we see the mental world as governed by free will. If we want to predict how something mechanical like a watch will behave, we need only know the laws that govern it. But when we make predictions about other minds, we assume they possess free will and are acting with intention. So how can we expect caregivers to suppress this powerful social instinct?

To do so might seem like a blessing. Yes, if we'd stop seeing intention, we wouldn't hold patients accountable and there would be fewer fights. On the other hand, we might be risking something far worse. When we no longer perceive intention, the regions of our brain engaged in social reasoning turn off, and we stop seeing people as having minds and devalue them as human beings. It's the neurological expression of "dehumanization," and not surprisingly, it has devastating consequences.

Months after Bartleby's death, the narrator hears a rumor that Bartleby had once been employed as a clerk in the Dead Letter Office, a government agency that disposes of undelivered letters addressed to people who are probably deceased. That Bartleby had worked in such a place must have deeply affected him, the narrator muses. After all, who wouldn't be depressed by all those letters that have nowhere to go? In other words, he's still trying to make sense of Bartleby's strange behavior. All of which leads me to a different understanding of Melville's final articulation: "Ah Bartleby! Ah humanity." It refers not only to the poor scrivener, as is commonly supposed, but also to the rest of us, those who do their utmost to grasp the incomprehensible.

Given the mind's egocentricity, it should not surprise us that people attribute more "human" qualities to themselves than to others. Empathy thus is accorded more to those we identify with than to those we find alien. Had the narrator come to accept Bartleby's mind as truly different from his own, his occasional impatience and anger might have been mitigated, but then his empathy would have been diminished as well. What continued to agitate our narrator was the same thing that compelled him to help and to feel that he could: the belief that he and Bartleby were essentially alike.

Caregivers face an analogous situation. They have to view patients as both sufficiently different from themselves, the better to stop perceiving intention, and yet sufficiently similar, so as not to lose sight of their humanity. It is a fine, nearly impossible, line to walk.

10

When the Right Thing Is the Wrong Thing

Why It's So Hard to Let Go of Blame

HAVING LED CAREGIVER SUPPORT GROUPS FOR TEN YEARS, I still feel a rush of gratitude and awe when members take a leap and reveal things they would not tell their closest friends. Group is the place where caregivers can find the understanding, compassion, and humor that elude them elsewhere, the place where they can openly grieve and even fall apart. Perhaps this exchange of trust between members never loses its poignancy for me because I know how delicate the process is and how quickly the feeling of safety can disappear.

I'm thinking specifically of a volatile thirty-five-year-old man—I'll call him James Hendley—who joined my older-adults group.* Although I worried that James might not be a good fit because he was younger than the others, I hoped that he would receive the support he desperately needed from more experienced caregivers. I also hoped that his vitriol and the intensity with which he expressed himself would give the members permission to access their own anger, which I had noticed this particular group was loath to do.

James was dealing with his mother, who generated in him enormous bitterness and hostility, feelings he readily shared. But instead of providing a catharsis, his anger only made the group feel trapped. Each time he raised his voice, the members tensed, shifted in their chairs, and looked away. Something about James's unhinged resentment and the repetitive loops of his tirades made sympathy difficult.

In his first meeting, the group learned that James's mother was nasty, mean, spiteful, and ungrateful. And that she liked playing mind games. This last grievance got the group's attention, and members wanted to hear more. So James recounted the time he had cooked a special dinner because his mother had asked for it. But when he served it, she had looked at the food contemptuously and said, "What is this?" James reminded her that she had requested the meal, but she denied doing so. And when he insisted that she eat it, she shoved the plate off the table.

"Do you see what I have to put up with?" James demanded.

---

* Nothing is more important than confidentiality in support groups since the purpose of the group is to encourage speech by ensuring privacy. Readers should be aware that I have taken pains to disguise the members. Despite such alterations, I have been faithful both to the emotions and the dynamic that so often emerge during group sessions.

But the group wasn't having it. Member after member reminded him (something I always discouraged) that it was memory loss, not mind games, that made her deny requesting the meal.

"I get that she has a disease, but why does she have to be so nasty about it?" James shouted.

Ordinarily, the group would have focused on the sadness beneath the theatrics, but James's truculent tone irritated them. It wasn't nastiness, members insisted, but mood swings, something his mother could not control.

"She was born with mood swings!" James retorted.

At this point, I interjected. I wanted the group to be less concerned about James's mother's emotional state and more about what it was doing to him. Not bothering to hide his satisfaction, James said he did not take his mother's abuse lying down. Whenever she pulled "one of her stunts," he called her out. He even told her that no one visited her because "no one wants to spend time with a nasty old woman."

When James finished, the oldest group member, Tom, spoke up. "You know," he said softly, "you'll never get the appreciation you want. It's just something you have to accept."

James glared at him, but Tom continued: "You have to understand that when your mom throws a tantrum, she's not responsible. She's sick, you're not, so it's you who has to stop playing games."

James fell silent, but in such a resentful way that he still managed to unsettle everyone. Perhaps Tom's quiet authority and his senior position in the group triggered something in the younger man. Usually when someone looks uncomfortable or reproachful, the others take a step back, allowing the person to recover his or her composure. Not this time. Instead, the members piled on, one after another, backing Tom's point of view.

The group's attitude was understandable, but I didn't like what was happening. The members were using James's intensity against him. But when I tried to redirect their attention, they were unresponsive. They remained fixated on James, one member even suggesting that he watch an educational video on dementia disorders.

"Okay," I said. "Enough. All this advice isn't helpful; it's not what we're here for. A lecture on Alzheimer's is not what James needs from us right now."

Taken aback, the group fell silent. I had never taken this tone before; I had never shot down something members had suggested.

Later, as I walked home, I chided myself. Ordinarily I would have allowed the group to explore what had happened. I'd have asked James what he was feeling when everyone was aligned against him, calling attention to how upsetting and dismissive the group's words must have felt. I would have urged the members to think about their need to "fix" James rather than simply listen to him. I had missed an opportunity to explore what James's anger toward his mother had brought out in the others.

By the time I reached my apartment some forty minutes later, I realized that I was actually angry, both at the group and at myself. I had done to them what they had done to James: I'd shut them down. It was the first time that I'd felt anything but affection for the group.

Although it might seem reasonable for the group to tell

James not to blame his mother for her behavior, I believe it is not only clinically damaging—that is, judgmental—but also too much to ask. By scolding James, the group dismissed (without knowing it) the very real vulnerabilities of the "healthy" brain that played such a large part in James's blaming his mother.

TO HELP US UNDERSTAND THE influences on our brain's moral reasoning, let's consider a classic thought experiment.

A runaway trolley is headed straight toward five people, all of whom will die if the trolley isn't stopped or diverted. You, however, have an opportunity to save them. By throwing a switch, you can direct the trolley onto another track, which will result in just one person's being killed.

What do you do? Most people do not hesitate to say they'd throw the switch.

Now consider another possibility: The same runaway trolley is again barreling toward five people, and the only way to save them is to physically push a sixth person off a footbridge so that his or her body will stop the trolley. Would you do it? Would you still sacrifice one life to save five?

Although it seems obvious that sacrificing one for many in the switch-throwing scenario is the right thing to do, the same decision feels morally wrong in the footbridge scenario. Why should this be the case if the end result is the same? A clue may be found in the neural correlates of each response.

In 2001, the philosopher and neuroscientist Joshua D. Greene and colleagues used an fMRI to observe what happens when people reason their way through certain moral dilemmas. In one such experiment, throwing the switch activated *cognitive* systems (including working memory and the dorsolateral, prefrontal, and parietal areas), while the footbridge scenario activated the *social/emotional* regions of the brain (the medial frontal gyrus, posterior cingulate gyrus, and bilateral superior temporal sulcus). Kant, who believed that emotions are separate from moral reasoning, would not have been pleased to learn the extent to which emotions come into play when making moral decisions.

Nonetheless, humans tend to be Kantian in this regard: Our intuitions—manifested in long-standing social and legal systems—embody the belief that moral judgments derive from an objective and "higher" reasoning. Guided by this belief, my group was convinced that James's emotions were preventing him from using reason to do the morally right thing. If only he could put his emotions aside, he'd be able to grasp that his mother's neural deficits were responsible for her "bad behavior." But this position ignores something fundamental. The latest research in affective neuroscience reveals that emotions don't just guide our automatic decisions; they are also essential in moral decision-making.

In point of fact, these decisions are not as "special" or "evolved" as we think. Drawing on Damasio's theory of somatic markers, the social psychologist Jonathan Haidt sets forth a "social intuitionist" model whereby emotions and their "automaticity"—i.e., their role in quick, intuitive, unconscious decisions—are actually *more* essential to moral decision-making than our slower, more deliberate cognition. This view is a bold rebuke to the traditional rationalist view of morality as a product of conscious, sophisticated reasoning—

what is often regarded as the most advanced stage in human development. The social intuitionist model posits that moral thinking is influenced by emotions and instincts, and only afterward does reason rationalize our emotion-fueled decisions. As Haidt eloquently puts it: "The emotions are, in fact, in charge of the temple of morality . . . moral reasoning is really just a servant masquerading as a high priest."

The idea that emotion accounts for our ethical and moral positions is hard to accept. But perhaps the primatologist Frans de Waal makes it easier to understand. De Waal takes a "bottom-up" approach to the subject, claiming that human morality evolves from the attachment systems common to all primates and mammals. This shouldn't surprise us, since biology is essentially economical in nature, and like many complicated processes, our moral sense piggybacks on existing mammalian responses. Feelings of right and wrong thus stem from the same innate and automatic instincts found in mammals. They, too, tend to favor cooperation and exhibit a proclivity for fairness, as well as disapproval of fellow mammals' social transgressions.

Even without possessing "higher reasoning," many mammals engage in complex interactions, abiding by an implicit social contract incorporating anger, gratitude, disgust, jealousy, joy, and fear. Indeed, animals even find ways to correct for behaviors that violate social norms, such as unfairness or lack of cooperation.

This doesn't mean that emotions are *always* at the helm of such decisions. Joshua D. Greene and others have argued for a "dual process" theory of morality, which holds that different scenarios influence the degree to which emotion or cognition comes into play. In situations that are felt as "personal"—such as physically shoving someone to his or her death—the *social/emotional* processing regions of the brain are activated, making it feel wrong to kill even if it's for the greater good. If, on the other hand, a moral dilemma does not feel personal—killing someone for the greater good simply by pulling a lever—the *cognitive* areas of the brain become activated, and killing becomes a calculation and therefore easier to justify.

You might wonder how this research is relevant to caregivers whose spouse or parent acts rudely or maliciously. Caregivers such as James will tell you that their family member's transgressions feel very personal. As we've seen, the closer we are to people, the more our social reasoning is "turned on" and the more we see their bad behavior as a moral violation. And how can a loved one's moral transgressions not feel personal?

To fully appreciate the caregiver's dilemma, we first have to acknowledge what's happening in the patient's brain. People with dementia are still capable of some moral reasoning and are very sensitive as to how they should be treated. They feel wronged if they regard themselves as slighted, rejected, or abandoned. James's mother, for example, judged him for misbehaving—while he, according to the group, was supposed to withhold moral judgment.

Put another way, James's inability to overlook his mother's violations issues from the "automaticity" of Kahneman's fast-thinking System 1. James may understand that his mother is sick, but conceptual awareness (System 2) cannot always hold back anger or judgment (System 1). Nonetheless, it seems reasonable to ask why James's "healthy" brain, whose executive function has not been impaired, is not capable of suppressing blame. The answer is that accepting a moral violation like unfairness takes a great deal of self-control, and self-control, as noted, is a limited resource. As dementia disorders inflict one injustice after another, caregivers carry an increasingly heavy cognitive load. In effect, James's own capacity for self-control has also been compromised.

We like to think that we judge a person's actions based on their mental state. Surely behavior that results from an accident or circumstances beyond a person's control ought to be considered before we judge her. But apparently human beings are not that fair-minded. When we feel a person's behavior is beyond the pale, judgment comes first. That is, we automatically tend to see intention in morally problematic behavior *whatever* the cause. How unfair, then, that caregivers are expected to resist seeing intention in the very behaviors that trigger this impulse.

In James's case, the group was simply responding in what it considered a reasonable manner: You can't blame a person if a disease is influencing her behavior. Without knowing it, the members were endorsing one side of a long-standing philosophical debate about determinism and moral responsibility. They intuitively took the "incompatibilist" position, which holds that people living in a deterministic world cannot be held morally responsible for their behavior. The "compatibilist" position, unintentionally represented by James, argues that free will and moral responsibility are separate and that the absence of the former does not absolve us of culpability. Although dementia disorders do not necessarily create a deterministic world for the patient, they can affect a patient's behavior, which is why the incompatibilist position seems to make more sense. Nonetheless, many caregivers like James continue to blame patients for behaviors they cannot control.

An experiment by the philosophers Shaun Nichols and Joshua Knobe sheds more light on why the group and James held different views. Nichols and Knobe created two hypothetical scenarios that test our intuitions about moral responsibility. In the first, or "abstract," situation, participants were instructed to read about a world where people's choices were predetermined. When asked if inhabitants of that world should be held morally accountable for their behavior, the participants almost unanimously took the incompatibilist view and replied "No."

Participants were then given a "concrete" scenario in which they were asked to imagine the same predetermined world but which now included a man named Bill. Bill had become infatuated with his secretary and decided that his wife and three children were obstacles to his happiness. So he torched his house, knowing that his family would die in the inferno. Deterministic world or not, participants found him morally responsible for what he did and condemned him for it.

Keeping in mind the first scenario, we easily understand the group's reaction to James. His mother, after all, was an abstraction, some older, vulnerable woman who lived in a universe where choice has been limited by Alzheimer's. But for James, his mother was as "concrete" as it gets, so he naturally took the compatibilist position and held her accountable.

The lesson to be drawn from Nichols and Knobe's two scenarios is that moral responsibility is defined less by how predetermined behavior is than by how we *feel* about that behavior. And because emotions play such an essential, albeit involuntary, role in our moral judgments, we're far more likely to accuse and punish when emotionally provoked by people. And who is better at provoking emotions than our family?

THINKING ABOUT THIS STUDY AND others like it, I wished the group had had a better understanding of what James's brain was up against. But would that necessarily have changed their minds? According to the philosopher Adina Roskies, advances in neuroscience and our increasingly mechanistic view of the brain will most likely not influence our moral views. An explicit knowledge of the brain's workings is no match for its intuitions, and some of our strongest intuitions involve the belief in free will and moral responsibility. At first, this might seem disheartening. Are we forever consigned to blame people, especially those close to us, no matter the reasons for their behavior?

In *The Ethical Brain,* Michael Gazzaniga views our instinct to hold others accountable in a different light. Unlike free will, Gazzaniga argues, moral accountability does not exist *in* the brain; it dwells between people, between minds. It is a communal trait built into society. Moral accountability, then, does not exist simply to assign blame. Accountability is an expectation we have of other minds; it's what gives them value while fostering reciprocity. As we saw in chapter 5, we associate people's "real" nature with their moral core. Thus, when we accept someone as no longer morally responsible, we tend to devalue that person as a human being.

This dehumanization, of course, is also one of the main goals of propaganda. As Paul Bloom asserts, propaganda is used to invalidate certain people's moral worth, making it easier to dismiss and dispose of them. Racist and anti-Semitic propaganda tropes have historically distorted human features in order to convey a brutish or animal-like appearance, thereby eliciting disgust. Disgust, Bloom says, is much more strategic than hate because it plays into mind-body intuitions, causing us to see another human being as a thing rather than a person with a mind. In effect, propaganda bypasses the social/emotional regions of the brain that help us feel moral responsibility toward other minds. And without this neural activation, there is no emotional distress when committing a personal violation.

When we stop seeing other minds as morally accountable, we risk dehumanizing them. What my support group missed, and what I also missed initially, was that James's unwillingness to stop blaming his mother was a way of reaffirming her moral standing. He wanted his mother to remain an ornery adversary, a woman who knew what she was doing. To accept something less, to accept that she was no longer morally accountable, would mean letting go of who she was. So at the same time that James was blaming his mother for this or that offense, he was also desperately holding on to her.

But why does holding on to someone necessarily mean assigning blame? The reason, again, is likely rooted in the intuition that people have a "good" deep-down self. This doesn't just include those we feel connected to; it also extends to those we deeply disagree with. And because we all define "good" based on our own values, James found it difficult to give up the idea that his mother might eventually come around to seeing his worth. His angry demands that she acknowledge his concern not only masked his vulnerability; it also contained a modicum of hope that one day he might reach the "real" her. It was a bitter, grudging hope, but hope nonetheless. And who are we to decide for James when he should let go of such hope?

ONE OF THE GREAT INJUSTICES of dementia disorders is that caregivers may have to renounce the implicit moral contract that exists between patients and themselves. At some point during the course of the disease, the patient's judgment becomes untrustworthy. This puts caregivers in an untenable position: In order to care for their patients, caregivers now have to make decisions for them, dissolving the moral context they once shared.

A caregiver I'll call Lila demonstrated this ethical tension. Lila came to see me about her best friend, Phillip. They were therapists who shared an office on the Upper West Side of Manhattan. Phillip was fifteen years older than Lila, and she considered him a friend and mentor. Not long after he turned sixty-five, Lila began to detect signs of early-to-middle-stage Alzheimer's. When she gently mentioned her concerns, Phillip dismissed them and refused to scale back his practice. This both worried and disappointed her. She thought treating patients in his condition was unethical. She knew, of course, that denial was often part of the disease, but that didn't make it any easier for her to accept his decision.

Although Phillip's impairment was obvious, Lila couldn't make herself believe that Alzheimer's had also affected his moral code. And though she was sure, as she told me, that "Phillip would be the first to say that a therapist should know when his emotional needs were getting in the way of the patient's well-being," she couldn't bring herself to intercede. True, she felt an ethical obligation both to Phillip and to his patients, but something held her back. For one thing, much of Phillip's clinical judgment remained intact, as did his sense of right and wrong. Indeed, he was still capable of offering Lila clinically sound advice about her own patients.

When I heard this, I explained that such expertise may last a long time and could be surprisingly nuanced. In other words, she should not be fooled by her friend's clinical abilities. But how could she make him quit? she wondered. We discussed whether she might float a white lie. She could pretend that Phillip's office needed to be fumigated, which meant that he would have to stop seeing patients for a while, during which time he might lose interest in practicing. But Lila didn't feel right about that. Not only would it prevent achieving closure with his patients, it would also ignore the fact that he had a problem.

I felt her discomfort. Phillip was still a clinician she admired, and if she lied, it would deny him the right to make decisions about his own career. By taking away this right, she would be, as Gazzaniga phrased it, "withdrawing [his] moral status."

So when do we need to accept that a parent, spouse, or friend is no longer morally accountable—that someone is no longer a person to be trusted to chose the right thing? It's an ethical dilemma bound to haunt caregivers and explains why, in many cases, caregivers wait too long before taking away driving privileges, or attaching a tracking device, or bringing an aide into the house. Safety matters, of course, but so does a person's integrity, which is tied to a feeling of autonomy. But in dealing with this disease, there is rarely a clear divide between right and wrong; there are only trade-offs. Even when we know our decisions are for the best, denying a person's right to choose still *feels* like a moral violation as long as we continue to see an essential moral self.

When Lila initially broached the subject to Phillip, she naturally hoped that he would scale back his practice. But her good intentions only caused a huge blowout, which upset them both. She was in a tough spot. As long as Phillip's moral reasoning was intact, what right did she have to make a moral decision for him? On the other hand, she had to consider the well-being of Phillip's patients. It isn't just denial or conflict aversion that causes caregivers to drag their feet about making these decisions. Such hesitation is part of the ambiguity involved in taking away a person's moral standing.

"He deserved to hear the truth," she said the second time we met.

I nodded but couldn't help wondering who, in this particular situation, really needed to hear the truth.

"If I were Phillip, I'd want to know," she insisted. "No matter how much it hurt, I'd need to know the reality."

Although I disagreed about confronting Phillip with the

extent of his cognitive decline, I couldn't blame her. Empathy, as we know, often begins with ourselves. We treat people the way we want to be treated, and Lila's feelings about Phillip were naturally bound up with her own sense of reality: She assumed that he required what she believed she'd want for herself.

Eventually Lila would stop regarding Phillip as a responsible moral agent, but she would have to come to it on her own. Nothing I could say would sway her, and why should it? In time Phillip would stop being a colleague altogether and become someone whose mind was failing. And Lila would have to redefine their relationship, readjust her expectations, and learn to live in *his* world as opposed to the one they used to share.

I knew this would happen because I had seen it many times in group. Not everyone gets there easily or quickly or completely. Support groups help not by educating but by allowing caregivers to feel what they're feeling, be it anger, fear, or sadness. Members bear witness to the impossible decisions they must make and give one another the emotional sustenance—and the permission—to make them. In a sense, the group becomes a surrogate for the person the caregiver is both looking after and slowly losing. And thus members allow one another to make moral decisions *with* rather than *for* others.

11

Word Girl

Why We Persist

WHEN PETER HARWELL'S SEVENTY-NINE-YEAR-OLD MOTHER punched a doctor in the face, Peter seemed to feel the impact himself. It was his aha moment: His mother had Alzheimer's. "It wasn't just a tap," Peter emphasized at our first meeting, but "an honest-to-God right hook." Shaken and embarrassed, he apologized to the doctor and hurried out of the office.

Once he and his mother were driving home, the world began to shift back to normal. "I did not like his tone and I did not care for his manner," his mother proclaimed. Tactfully, Peter conceded there had been a strange edge to the doctor's request that she undress. "Damn right there was," she retorted. She then launched into one of her rants about the medical profession, and with every word and every mile, Peter felt further and further removed from his moment of clarity. How could his mother have Alzheimer's when she spoke so incisively?

Peter and his mother shared a passion for words: puns, puzzles, offbeat expressions, wordplay, and banter. He called her his Word Girl, and in a professional sense that's exactly what she was. Mary Harwell had been a respected journalist and later a star in the advertising world when both professions had been dominated by men. But she had easily held her own, disarming and impressing her male colleagues because, as Peter fondly explained, "Mom was a verbal gunslinger." She cursed like a sailor, she liked a good joke, she was quick on the uptake and quick with a barb, and she had an unbeatable work ethic. And woe to anyone who disrespected her. She had no compunction about verbally eviscerating those who got out of line.

People who knew Mary were not surprised by what had happened at the doctor's office. When Mary was a little girl in New Jersey, her mother had needlessly dragged her to doctors' offices. Her father didn't want his wife to work, and with nothing to do, she began to obsess over real and imaginary ailments. As soon as Mary got her period, her mother took her to an OB-GYN. They showed up without an appointment and were told the doctor couldn't see them. But Mary's mother made a scene and refused to leave. After a long wait the doctor appeared. He told Mary's mother to stay outside while he examined Mary. The doctor then proceeded to molest her. When Mary yelled that he was hurting her, the doctor berated her for wasting his time. Later they learned that he had a reputation for sexually assaulting the daughters of immigrants because he knew the parents wouldn't lodge a complaint.

Twenty years later, Mary was assaulted again, this time in her own home while her husband was away. When she reported the rape to the police, she was told there was no evidence and that she was lucky that it hadn't been worse. Feeling dismissed for the second time, she stopped trusting the police—or anyone else who was supposed to protect her.

Forty-six years later, when she delivered a right hook to the doctor's jaw, Peter's first thought was Alzheimer's—but was it? Neither Peter nor his father could rule out the possibility that her past history had been a contributing factor. The difference between dementia disorders and preexisting PTSD is often subtle; both conditions cause patients to misread cues and overreact to nonthreatening events. In fact, many preexisting disorders can mirror, disguise, or exaggerate dementia symptoms, making it difficult to notice the emergence of a new pathology.

Because of Mary's history, Peter and his father weren't sure what to think even after she was diagnosed. Usually they underplayed her disease, leaning on what Peter referred to as the family's "lubrication of the day," the process of reducing friction with conversation, good manners, and humor. Indeed, whenever Mary became emotionally volatile, Peter and his father would tease her for being a "Celtic storm," which always made her laugh, and her willingness to laugh at herself made them think she was still her old self. Although proud of his family's tact and ability to deflect, Peter also knew it could be a drawback.

"It's a good way to live," Peter told me, adding wistfully, "but not so good when it comes to recognizing dementia."

"In what way?" I asked.

"Oh, you know. When Mom said she was going gaga, Dad and I would chime in with, 'You're not the only one. We're all going downhill, we're always forgetting stuff.'"

"It's funny," Peter observed, "when you keep comforting someone enough, saying the same thing over and over, those words kind of become you. You believe it yourself."

In repose, Peter had a dignified, handsome face, which on closer inspection looked exhausted from decades of caregiving—first for his father and now for his mother. He had sharp features, sunken cheeks, gray hair, and thoughtful gray eyes. It was a good, arresting face, and I wasn't surprised to learn that he had acted off-Broadway and done commercials and voiceovers before becoming a caregiver. His voice was deep and expressive, and once he started speaking, his face softened and became animated as his mind darted from one subject to another. An inveterate theatergoer, voracious reader, and movie buff, Peter tended to pile on references and often apologized for his copious allusions. But I loved listening to him, because more than anyone else I knew, he took pleasure in talking.

"It's in my genes," he said half-seriously.

Mary's affinity for words had, of course, led to her storied career. She was considered a female pioneer in the advertising world but had no patience for accolades. She was, she liked to say, just a girl who liked spy novels, chitchatting, and throwing ideas around. And according to Peter that hadn't changed much with the advent of dementia. Mary could still command a room with her conversation, and so, despite her glitches, odd behavior, and forgetfulness, Peter sometimes found it hard to accept that his mother was truly ill.

AFTER PETER'S FATHER DIED, MARY'S condition deteriorated. Dementia made her more sensitive than ever to any sign that her competence or independence was being questioned. The more she needed help, the more she resisted it. Making sure that she was safe while also allowing her to feel in control became a tricky balancing act for Peter. Bath time was the worst. She gradually lost interest in showering and developed infections under her breasts and in her urinary tract, which led to psychosis and trips to the hospital. Even when she did shower, she might forget to use soap. Peter then had to help her.

"I don't mean to be indelicate," he told me uncomfortably, "but washing your mother, to do it effectively, you have to touch her in places that, you know, you touch someone when you're being intimate."

"I cannot imagine how difficult that must have been," I said.

"It was awful for both of us, but I tried to be objective about it. I have this mantra: 'It's just matter. We're all matter. I'm just doing a job.'"

The mantra came in handy when his mother would yell, "Let go of me, you son of a bitch! What do you think you're doing? Let go or I'll call the police."

Peter hated seeing his mother—a formidable, brilliant, self-reliant woman—in such a helpless state. He felt he was denying her the right to make decisions about her own body, and when she yelled at him, he detected in her voice not just rage, but also the unresolved trauma of being attacked by someone she had trusted. It was awful that he was now that someone.

"Did you ever consider hiring some professional help?" I asked. "A female aide?"

The question actually caused him to blanch. "I tried it and it was a disaster. She wouldn't stand for it."

In fact, his mother was so furious the one time a stranger had tried to help her undress that Peter became afraid for the aide's safety. One wrong move and it would be the doctor's office all over again.

"I suppose I could have given it another try," he said doubtfully, "but I just couldn't. My mother angry is just something I can't take."

I nodded. Many caregivers avoid getting professional help for one reason or another, but I suspected that in Peter's case it wasn't Mary's anger that stopped him, but his own fear that he would be re-traumatizing her. He had clearly internalized her two assaults and couldn't bear to put her in an unpredictable situation again.

Unfortunately, with a disease like Alzheimer's, anything a caregiver chooses to do has the potential to feel like a betrayal. Unwilling to cause his mother more pain by bringing in an aide, Peter learned to power through those long minutes when he helped her shower. He'd distract her with silly lines from James Bond movies or with the promise of watching a favorite John Ford western. On good days he worked fast, and before she realized it he had lifted her breasts and applied her ointment. On other days he noticed that just as she was about to lunge at him, a visceral animal awareness made her sense that she was actually being cared for (perhaps because the ointment felt good against her skin). In any case, her mood would lighten, and she'd say, "You're good to me, Peter, you're good to me."

I commended Peter for how well he handled this terribly awkward task, but Peter waved the compliment off. "You know, for a long time—decades, actually—I drank, and let's say I made some mistakes. But being there for my mom, it's not even a question. It's what she deserves. I put my parents through the wringer, and I'm glad I can pay them back in some small way. It's not why I do it, but I'm honored that I get the chance."

Noticing how touched I was, he instinctively tried to deflect my admiration. He wasn't always patient, he allowed. It depended on which Mary he was dealing with. Some days his mother was "evil incarnate." And he always knew it would be a bad day when instead of removing her robe she'd give him one of her trademark sneers: "What are you, strange? You want to see your mother naked?" The fact that this scene had already played out a hundred times made no difference, since she retained no memory of it.

"You think I want to see you naked?" he'd retort. "You're not exactly Ursula Andress, you know."

"I just showered," she'd insist.

"It's been a week, and we have to worry about infections."

"No, I showered yesterday!"

"You didn't. You don't remember things now."

"Who says?"

"The doctor."

"Let me call that son of a bitch!"

"Mom, remember you ended up going to the hospital? Remember how miserable you were?"

"Oh, I remember," she chortled. "You wanted to lock me up in that shithole and take all my money. And everyone thought you were such a good son!"

"You gave me no choice! You were sick."

His mother had eyed him suspiciously. "I know you, little man. You've got others fooled, but not me. You are a 'house devil, town saint.'"

This old Irish expression of hers usually delighted him, but not now. He was tired of being demeaned, and infuriated by the accusation that he was after her money.

"Listen here, you better shut the fuck up because you don't know what the hell you're talking about. You think I want to do this?"

"I know you," his mother replied. "You're a failure. You've always been a failure. You've done nothing. I . . . I *did* things."

When Peter saw my pained reaction, he gave me a resigned smile: "Oh, she knows how to get you where it hurts. And I'm going to be honest. At that moment I wanted to hurt her. I mean, I wanted to choke her right there and then."

He glanced at me, wondering whether I was shocked by

his confession—probably because he felt shocked by it himself.

But I simply told him the truth: "All that time alone with your mother and no one helping you or giving you a break, I can't imagine that you could feel anything else. So what did you do?"

"I grabbed her by the shoulders, but then I stopped. I went to another part of the house. I texted a friend. I breathed."

I was relieved, as much for Peter as for Mary. Everyone knows that living with dementia is difficult, but most people don't know that it can bring out new and unwelcome aspects of yourself.

"You did good, Peter," I murmured. "You stepped away when it mattered."

MARY AND PETER HAD FIRST started ice skating together as a lark. Neither one was any good, but it was something they could do together, and they enjoyed observing and listening to the other skaters as they went around and around. No snippet of conversation was too small to report back to Peter's father and dissect. But when his father was struggling with cancer, they stopped going to the rink. His father insisted, of course, that they get their skates and "skedaddle," but Mary was adamant. She was too loyal, too stubborn.

These characteristics which Peter so admired later challenged him after she developed Alzheimer's. Her intractability increased with her confusion and anxiety, and it often made caring for her next to impossible. Day after day, he encountered more resistance to the showering. Day after day, he had to argue, threaten, and cajole before she would consent. Then, on one occasion, Mary surprised him: first docilely removing her robe, then standing defiantly naked and declaring through clenched teeth: "I am not taking your goddamn shower."

Seeing his mother naked, vulnerable, yet utterly unmovable filled Peter with unbearable sadness. He didn't have it in him to see his mother in pain. He didn't have it in him to take her to the hospital again. Why did she have to resist? Why did he have to go through this every time? "Do it for me," he begged.

This only irritated her. "What are you, strange?" she taunted. "A strange boy who wants to shower his mother? To see his mother naked?"

Unhinged, he fell on his knees and violently shook his head.

Seeing him on all fours, Mary became confused. "What the hell are you doing?" she said. "Get up! Get up!"

But he was in the grip of his own misery. Suddenly he took off his glasses and to his own amazement crushed them in his hands. With bleeding palms he lifted the shattered frame like a sacrificial offering. He didn't know why he'd crushed his glasses. Perhaps because he couldn't hurt his mother, he hurt himself. Perhaps he simply wanted to shock her. Or perhaps by breaking his glasses, he wanted to break the repetitive loop they were trapped in.

His mother had looked at him with a mixture of pity and impatience. "Do I need to call the cops?"

Recalling the incident for me, Peter began to laugh, a semi-hysterical laugh that I had heard from other caregivers. It occurred to him how absurd he must have looked. His mother had already moved on from the drama of showering and had probably forgotten she was naked. All she knew at that moment was that her son was on the floor groveling, his hands bleeding for no discernible reason.

"Peter," she had said, sternly but not unkindly, "have you lost your mind?"

This seemed possible to him. The repetition, the anxiety, the same senseless accusations had simply become too much. Then he noticed Mary's robe lying a few feet away, the leopard robe she always wore. *How dirty it must be,* he thought. Every day he wanted to throw it into the washing machine, and every day he ended up not doing it because he knew it would upset her. He picked up the robe and helped her slip into it. He suggested they order pizza and watch a movie. She immediately brightened. A half hour later the pizza arrived and Mary was content, humming along to the opening credits of a Bond film. But while Mary quickly became engrossed in the silly plot, Peter was still shaken. He couldn't stop thinking that he had failed "as a son and as a person."

I ALWAYS LOOKED FORWARD TO seeing Peter because I never knew where our talks would lead. What I did know was that his humor, animated soliloquies, sudden digressions, and just as sudden return to the main thread belied his mental and physical exhaustion. Some days I sensed were worse than others, days when Peter's thoughts turned to how his father might have dealt with the disease. One particular image stayed with him: his father perched on the kitchen counter, half reading the newspaper and half listening to Peter trying to convince his mother of something. Usually he didn't meddle, but one day, after another argument had reached a crescendo, he lowered his newspaper and said gently but firmly, "Peter, why do you *bother*?"

Peter looked at him, unsure how to respond.

His father looked calmly back and said: "I know you and Mom have this verbal thing going, but you're driving yourself crazy. It's not good for you, son."

Years later, Peter still felt he was letting his father down. Although I pointed out that his father had had a son to lean on whereas Peter was dealing alone with a progressive disease, the question nagged at him: "Why do you bother?" By now, Peter figured, he should have learned to stop. But what is true in life becomes even more true with dementia: We get drawn into meaningless arguments even though we know they'll lead nowhere. And it isn't just a patient's habitual behaviors or our own philosophical intuitions or the function of the left-brain interpreter that creates the itch to argue. The cause is something so simple that we overlook it: conversation itself.

The cognitive psychologists Simon Garrod and Martin J. Pickering maintain that conversation is deceptively "easy"—an observation that until quite recently went against the academic grain. Most cognitive scientists believed that speaking and listening were relatively simple operations while conversation was complex—complex because it was often unplanned and fragmentary, necessitating a back-and-forth between listening and speaking.

But Garrod and Pickering take a different tack: Conversation is difficult only if we presume that the listener and the speaker are independent entities, constituting two distinct neural processes. Of course, this is exactly how conversation was perceived as long as the production of speech and the comprehension of speech were viewed as separate cognitive events—to be studied in isolation and only in labs.

Although the research is still relatively new, an alternative theory has emerged that considers listening and talking as a *joint* activity in which "interactive alignment" creates a "perceptual-behavioral expressway" between two people. Just as our motor neurons mirror someone picking up a cup of coffee as though we're picking it up ourselves, a speaker and listener imitate each other. The listener's brain represents what the speaker is saying as though she were uttering the same words, and the better the listener and speaker understand each other, the more intimately their brains engage in "neural coupling"—i.e., exhibiting the same representations in the auditory or motor regions of the brain. Moreover, there is lots of overlap in the cognitive regions responsible for beliefs, intention, and meaning.

According to Garrod and Pickering, conversation is a collaborative activity, a co-construction, so to speak, with each person simulating the grammar, vocabulary, and tone of the other. As in riding a seesaw, the momentum that each person generates helps propel the other. This is what psychologists mean by "cognitive ease." Conversation is easy because once initiated, it continues automatically, requiring neither deliberation nor conscious control. And, as we have seen again and again, our brain is strategically lazy; it loves to save energy. Dementia or no dementia, engaging in conversation is a neural habit that is very hard to resist.

As conversations continue to unfold, they also become easier because verbal options become more limited. When we automatically "borrow" from the person we're speaking to, our lexical paths narrow. Instead of having to sort through hundreds of choices about which words to use or what grammatical structures best frame our thoughts, we are guided by our companion's speech. This naturally requires less cognitive energy than, say, following instructions, which is why dementia patients are more capable of arguing with us about what we say than they are of actually doing what we ask.

Because conversation is by definition social, dementia patients remain capable of verbally interacting with others long after their other faculties begin to deteriorate. Indeed, one reason Mary slipped so naturally into her role as Word Girl is that conversation gave her a cognitive boost. In time, the disease may sharply curtail verbal facility, and caregivers often end up carrying on "conversations" by themselves. This is not only psychologically painful, another way of losing a loved one; it's also cognitively draining. But as long as patients piggyback on what others say, caregivers continue to believe that they and their parent or spouse are on the same cognitive page.

AS WE SAW IN CHAPTER 6, we invariably overestimate the degree to which other minds see the world as we do, and con-

versation only perpetuates this misconception. Like everything having to do with the brain's evolution, conversation is,
in a sense, all about prediction. In fact, our minds try to imitate other minds in order to help make such predictions. And
to make reasonable guesses about the people we're talking to,
we assume that their brain is pretty much like our own. Even
if the other person has cognitive issues, we unconsciously
make predictions based on the assumption that our brains
remain very much alike.

Although caregivers know that patients suffer from a
dementia disorder, as soon as they hear the familiar protests
and accusations, their brains unwittingly begin to meld with
the patients'. Two brains then automatically start to imitate
each other, bait each other, and tantalizingly create the illusion that true understanding is within reach.

Complicating matters further, as patients become
increasingly untethered, their words still imply a shared history. When Mary Harwell felt that Peter was after her money
and wanted to send her off to a nursing home, she went on
the offensive, repeating "I know you, you're nothing. You did
nothing. *I* did things." And though Peter knew that she was
sick, her words hurt because they evoked a mutual past, a
past now being used against him.

"It hurt because she wasn't really wrong," Peter confessed
at one of our last meetings. "She actually did something. She
became somebody, a success. Me, I'm not exactly viable. I
mean, I had to care for my dad and then my mom, and I'd do
it again and again. But I can't say I've done much with my
life."

Hearing Peter speak about himself in this way was deeply

upsetting. How could his mother use her son's sacrifice against him? Didn't she know that his professional life never took off because he had to take care of his parents for over twenty years? Couldn't she understand that he was her sole protector, doing everything he could to make her life better? Then I caught myself. Of course she didn't know; she had Alzheimer's.

Nonetheless, like Peter during one of his frequent arguments with Mary, I could not help but hold her words against her.

WORDS, AS EVERY CAREGIVER LEARNS eventually, become meaningless—not merely because they'll soon be forgotten, but also because grammar, which fixes and frames words, doesn't align with the realities of dementia. Grammar, as Nietzsche pointed out, both guides and restricts us. When we say "The lightning flashed," Nietzsche cautioned, it sounds as though something is lighting up the sky. But lightning cannot flash; the lightning *is* the flash. Because of how words and syntax work, we always assume agency, a doer, someone or something that *chooses* to act. It's a fallacy that has practical consequences for caregivers, since we tend to see intention even where none exists. Language is just one more way of demonstrating this intuition.

According to the philosopher Patrick Haggard, language inadvertently confirms the mind-body intuition because "it always implies a mental 'I' as distinct from both the brain and the body." This "I" we feel chooses to say or do things. So when someone uses "I" we immediately hear intention. When patients shout "I won't do this" or "I don't want that," we hear presence of mind, a consciousness that knows what it wants. Even when patients lament that their brains "don't work," it only adds to the impression that their minds still do.

In effect, we tend to hear speech as the product of a disembodied mind, a phenomenon not subject to the body's whims and weaknesses. And when words are deployed in a sophisticated manner, it makes us even more convinced that the speaker is "still in there." So when Mary said, "I don't need a shower," Peter perceived not only intention, but also a unified self. Hearing that pronoun, he automatically heard his Word Girl rather than a neurological illness. Her words alone made him forget that ten minutes later she would not remember them.

It's not only a patient's words that fool us. When I hear caregivers describe family members as "selfish," "stubborn," "lazy," "obstinate," or "mean," it doesn't occur to me that they are being unkind or unaware of the disease. Instead I am reminded that there are really no words that represent a neurological source of a patient's behavior. We only have psychological descriptions.

Built into language—its logic and structure—are intuitions that make us feel that the speaker's memory is intact. Verb tenses, for instance, necessarily project a sense of time. When patients say, "I'll do it later" or "I promise I won't touch the stove," they fool both themselves and others into believing they can remember. By promising, threatening, or reassuring us, spouses and parents can make us feel that we're still moving together in time. And because the logic of "if X, then Y" continues to be part of their linguistic repertoire, we actually expect them to follow through.

Whenever Peter and his mother argued, part of him believed that if he just found the right words, his mother would understand and everything could be resolved. She'd do what he asked, and she wouldn't berate him for trying to help her. Hope followed by disappointment becomes its own tedium. But, as Peter explained, the day-to-day drudgery of searching for solutions becomes so ingrained that one doesn't realize that nothing ever gets accomplished.

"Before you know it," he said, "ten years have gone by and you wonder, 'What happened? Where did the time go?'"

In that moment, as we sat in my office on a cool spring day, it occurred to me that while Peter was trying to impose his sense of time on Mary, he had in actuality inherited his mother's timelessness. Because time did not really exist for Mary and she was essentially the only person Peter ever saw, time had become less real for him as well. Mother and son now existed in a state of perpetual sameness. Every day the same routines, the same arguments. How did they fill the timelessness? With conversation—and conversation, no matter how haphazard or disjointed, still held for him the possibility of change.

He paused and then asked if I had ever read *Waiting for Godot*. I nodded (perhaps too vigorously) because it's a play I had often thought about during my time in the Bronx.

"When you think about it," Peter said, "all that happens in the play is talk. That's what the characters do, they talk.

The dialogue is ridiculous, it's fragmentary, but when you take it all in, the totality of it all, it starts to sound normal."

I agreed and urged him to continue.

"Ah, I'm just riffing," he said apologetically. "You know my mom would mock me for talking this way. She'd call me out and say I was being pretentious and maybe I am . . ." He trailed off, but then picked up with renewed energy. "See, the conversations might seem inane, but they work because the words feed off each other. Kind of like my mom and me. A lot of what goes on with us is ridiculous, but it also makes sense because it feels like at least we're doing *something*. It may just be empty calories filling you up without being nourishing, but they provide just enough energy to keep you going. Does that make any sense?"

It did make sense. *Waiting for Godot* is a play seemingly about two down-and-out characters, Vladimir and Estragon, who are waiting for someone named Godot. The play ripples with nonsensical misunderstandings, pointless quibbles, inconsequential mutterings, illogical arguments, empty promises, and empty threats, all of which end at night and start up again the next day. Both characters believe that as soon as Godot comes, everything will change.

While they wait, nothing much happens. The audience observes the two oddballs standing aimlessly, obsessing over the fit of shoes, the position of a tree, or which is the tastier end of a carrot. And, as if anticipating the audience's impatience, Vladimir quips, "This is becoming really insignificant." Yet they go on as before, and this pointless going on is, I suspected, what Peter related to. Vladimir and Estragon sustain themselves by conversing, by using language to both characterize and ward off the meaninglessness of their existence. It was not the hope of Godot's arrival that kept them going, but the hope that is built into the fabric of language.

"As long as we have faith in grammar," Nietzsche observed, "we cannot rid ourselves of God." What he meant, I think, is that even hardened atheists implicitly believe in some greater order because syntax itself presupposes agency and meaning. When communicating, we partially redress whatever chaos, unpredictability, and unruliness exist around us.

All conversation is, in a sense, hopeful. By conversing, we create and acknowledge the possibility that clarity, meaning, and connection exist even when there appears to be only strangeness and futility. And this is what Beckett understood: Language creates absurdity but also protects us from it. Even when Vladimir and Estragon grumble about the pointlessness and emptiness of communication, they're still communicating. Talking carries them along, it gives them something to do, and before they know it, dusk has fallen. As Peter had observed, conversation acts as a lubricant, allowing one day to slide into the next. It may not seem like much, but as long as we converse, we can hope, even if it's a resigned, almost oppressive hope.

THE NEXT TIME PETER CAME to see me, he told me that he couldn't get *Godot* out of his mind. He thought he now understood how Mary had sucked him into those meaningless confrontations. It wasn't just the idioms and phrases that she used; she also *sounded* like Mom. Even her incoherent mutterings possessed a familiar musical quality. So when Peter spoke to her, he was, in a manner of speaking, carrying a tune that he had hummed innumerable times before.

As I listened to Peter, a thought began to form: The reason the nutty, obscure, and flamboyant conversations in *Godot* feel eerily familiar is that the music of the sentences draws us in and, without our knowing it, makes us identify with the characters. We accept their aggravation, their obsessions, their misery, their imaginative leaps, as well as their inability to part from each other despite the constant threats to do so. In effect, the rhythm of their words becomes the rhythm of life, and we all too easily fall under its spell.

And this led me to wonder if the often combative dynamic between patient and caregiver isn't also facilitated by something more than the cognitive ease built into conversation. Maybe the dynamic also proceeds from the *sound* of language, a sonority that lures us into further conversations. Music, as we know, has the uncanny ability to reawaken patients with neurological disorders, igniting parts of the mind believed to be gone. Could not, then, the familiar rhythms and inflections of conversation also coax a dementia patient back to a reality they once shared with someone?

Peter and his mother had a comedy routine they often performed. One would pretend to desperately want something—a book, a piece of candy, a cup of coffee, it didn't matter—and incessantly plead for it. The other then pretended to become outraged and hotly refused the request. Although the origins of the joke were now obscure, the interplay, the act itself, remained fresh. So when his mom was feeling low, Peter might suddenly adopt a wheedling tone and say, "Mom, can

I please, *pleeese* have a cookie?" Hearing this, Mary would immediately respond indignantly, "No, no, no, you cannot have a cookie!" Both would then dissolve into helpless laughter.

Even after Mary had had dementia for years, the shtick still worked. One of the last times I saw Peter, a few weeks after Mary's death, he recalled a time when he'd visited his mother in hospice. He had found Mary in a weakened, almost somnolent state, unable to reply to his questions with anything but a weary yes or no. At one point, however, she softly asked Peter to hand her the glass of water standing on the bedside table. "No!" Peter suddenly shouted to the horrified amazement of the nurses and visitors nearby. "You cannot have a glass of water. No water for you!" Immediately Mary knew what was up and gleefully began to beg for the water. "Please, pleeese, water. Water, pleeeese." The more she begged, the harsher his refusals—until once again, as always, they collapsed, shrieking with laughter.

And at that moment, Peter felt that he had gotten his Word Girl back, the woman who teased and loved being teased. "Now, that's really Mom," he said.

And what happens when it is all over, when both the disease and the patient are gone? Can caregivers resume their former lives and pick up where they left off? Of course, this is exactly what bereaved caregivers are encouraged to do. Friends and relatives, who seem as uncomfortable around the pain of grief as around the heartache of caregiving, tell them, "It's time to move on." They want caregivers to feel a sense of relief now that the ordeal is over. Some manage to do this; others find it more difficult.

When I run into caregivers whose partner or parent has passed away, I usually know before they tell me. Something is different about them. Yes, they seem more rested and no longer have the tense, haunted look of people anticipating a crisis, but something seems amiss. One day a former caregiver admitted that although he was no longer coping with the stress of caregiving, he was struggling "to adjust to real life." That was it, I thought: There's an indefinable feeling of aimlessness about a bereft caregiver, an uncertainty about the future and one's place in it.

Having spent so much time adjusting to a loved one's reality, accommodating another person's logic, and constantly responding to his or her needs, a former caregiver can find life after a patient's death to be almost as foreign as Alzheimer's itself. Many can scarcely wrap their minds around the idea that from minute to minute, nothing is expected of them. Nor is it only their minds that struggle to adjust; a phantom adrenaline seems to course through their bodies—but to what end?

Stress remains, but it's the ordinary, protracted kind: unpaid medical bills, houses and apartments in shambles, clothing and furniture that need disposing of, as well as health issues of their own after years of neglect. The untapped energy or anxiety, however, resides elsewhere. Some people find that they have been hiding behind their patient's needs. Indeed, what had once oppressed them also helped to define them. Who are they now with no one to look after?

Whatever their past or current discomfort, many claim they would do it all over again, and almost all feel compelled to add, "But this time I would do it differently." Indeed, their biggest regrets tend to center on their own behavior. Why had they engaged in fighting? Resorted to harsh words? Shown such inflexibility? Adjusted so slowly to the disease in all its stages? Hearing them express remorse, I imagine their minds as echo chambers of self-recrimination, tolling their failings as caregivers, as children and spouses, as human beings.

But I suppress the urge to interrupt. I don't want them to

beat themselves up. I've spoken to too many caregivers not to recognize the real culprit behind their "bad" behavior. So I keep quiet. Words of comfort are not what they need from me. What they need is to voice their regrets. And if I have learned anything, it is that evidence, no matter how obvious or logical, usually does not change people's feelings—not for long, anyway—and certainly not before they're ready to change.

WHEN I BEGAN WRITING THIS book, I wanted to better understand the difficulties caregivers contend with, especially the self-inflicted kind: the self-flagellation, the seemingly irrational behavior, and the remorse that follows. And because these reactions seem almost universal, I sensed that something more than impatience and frustration was at work.

Indeed, the more I listened to caregivers and the more I read about the brain, the more it occurred to me that the "healthy" brain's ingrained biases and proclivities make it unequipped in many ways to deal with the cognitively impaired brain. Because of such neurological constraints, I wanted caregivers to understand that it was not character flaws that made caregiving so fraught, but rather their own brain's intrinsic workings. And naturally I hoped they would accord themselves the same forgiveness that they're encouraged to offer their patients.

Having said this, it would be naïve to think that caregivers or, for that matter, anyone reading this book will absolve themselves of culpability for their actions because they understand the neurological reasons behind them. After all, we're inclined and perhaps conditioned to believe that our neural networks do not define us: That we're in charge of our actions. That we decide what is right and wrong. We struggle to accept the idea that moral transgressions have a neurological source. And because we feel this way, we have trouble forgiving loved ones for their behavior despite our awareness of *their* brain's deficits.

I still remember how discouraged I was after I showed Sam photographs of the "Alzheimer's brain." Looking at the pictures, he saw that the problem was his father's brain, not his personality, but the realization kept his temper in check for only an hour or two before their old contentious dynamic resumed. Similarly, when I presented Sam with evidence (during the course of writing this book) that his own brain had inevitably reacted to his father's Alzheimer's with its own set of neural responses, he took some comfort in the fact that his behavior was hardly unique—and yet this feeling, too, didn't last. Before long he again felt that the mistakes he made were *his* and not the product of his brain's circuitry.

I'm no different from other former caregivers. When I think back on my time in the Bronx, I continue to reprimand myself: "If I could do it again, I wouldn't make the same mistakes. This time I'd get it right." And though I've written a book about what the healthy brain is up against when dealing with a diseased brain, I still cannot quite accept the fact that the brain's limitations are *my* limitations.

And perhaps that's all right. As Kahneman likes to remind us, the biases and tendencies that make us fallible are also what make the mind a marvel. The intuitions that make it so hard to see and accept the disease are the *same* intuitions that allow us to feel connected to the person whose mind is irreparably changing. The intuitions that make us blame vulnerable patients also help us feel a deep moral accountability to them. And the intuitions that make it hard to let go of our hurt and anger also help us hold on to a patient's humanity. Nothing about how our minds work is inherently one thing or another, and neither are we.

I hope that current and former caregivers may all come to see this, but the realizations must arrive on a timeline unique to every person, and it's not for me or anyone else to shorten it. Years ago, I did my best to change a caregiver's self-sabotaging behavior and assuage the guilt that followed. Now, however, I believe our efforts should be directed elsewhere. I believe that dementia disorders and perhaps life itself are best approached not by trying to change minds or challenging another person's reality, but by striving to understand a mind, to see it in context, to reckon with its contradictions, and simply to let *that* mind know it is worth knowing.

Acknowledgments

There are many people to thank. First, all the caregivers who spoke to me and gave me so much of their time. Of course, I'm particularly indebted to those caregivers who fill the pages of this book. They moved me not only by their love and sacrifice but by their unflinching honesty about the toll of caregiving. They offered me their experiences so that other caregivers, reading this, might feel less alone.

I also want to thank my first case study, Sam K., who wasn't just kind enough to allow me to use his story but insisted that I do so. Without his encouragement to write down my thoughts, and his belief that there was something to write about, I would not have taken the leap.

So much changed for me when I met James Marcus. His generosity and guidance were both immensely helpful. He gave me the benefit of his friendship, for which I am most grateful.

My good fortune continued when James introduced me to my thoughtful, caring, and protective agent, Jin Auh. After reading an essay and a short proposal, she immediately grasped the story I wanted to tell and the urgency I felt to tell it. It was Jin's acumen and intuition that led her to the ideal editor for my book. That would be Hilary Redmon, and I cannot imagine having a more sensitive and discerning editor. Hilary didn't just give shape to an unwieldy manuscript, she revealed to me what my book could and should become. She also happens to be a joy to work with.

Before there was a book, there was an essay, and I am grateful to Robert Wilson for accepting my essay in *The American Scholar,* and to Sudip Bose for his kindness and astute edits.

For decades Jed Levine has been a source of knowledge about dementia disorders, but it is his thoughtfulness and sensitivity that has garnered him the trust of so many families. The fact that he trusted me with some of their stories means more than I can say.

Abby Nathanson had confidence in my clinical abilities, and I owe to her the privilege of working with many caregivers and especially with support group leaders, some of the most insightful and generous people I have ever met.

And thank you to Marilucy Lopes, who walked me through some difficult situations and whose warmth, humor, and wise counsel make everything easier.

Because Yaddo gave me a place to think, swim, and feel cared for, my book was finally able to coalesce.

The Society Library and the people who work there made the formidable task of writing feel slightly less daunting.

I also wish to thank my early readers Pamela Dailey and Kerry Fried for their feedback at a crucial time, and Jonathan

Galassi for his faith in my book and for his letters of recommendation.

My thanks also go out to Joshua Knobe, Michael Gazzaniga, and Daniel Schacter for their close reading of various chapters of the manuscript.

And a special thank-you to Norman Doidge, whose kindness and perspicacity, not to mention the time and effort he invested, came just when I needed it.

I am very fortunate to have a loving brother in Dmitry (Dima) Kiper, whose willingness to help is matched only by his ability to do so.

Then there are my old friends, whose support and general delight in the prospect of this book helped sustain me: Inna Buschell, Alisa Curley, and Marina Flider.

I'd also like to thank Arthur Krystal, my friend.

Finally, there are my parents, Masha (Mariya) and Alex Kiper, to whom I dedicate this book. Their love and kindness made everything possible.

Below are a few recommendations to help you gather some resources and support as a dementia caregiver. The list is not exhaustive, and many of these recommendations provide similar services and address similar issues. The goal is to find an organization, an author, or a resource that is the right fit for you. And since every caregiver, every family, every person living with dementia (PLWD) is different, none of these recommendations are going to be right for everyone. When it comes to knowing and understanding your and your family's needs, you, the reader, are the expert.

Also, because a caregiver's to-do list can seem never-ending, try tackling only a few things at a time. You can't do it all, and you can't do it all alone. Which is why I recommend paying just as much attention to resources that can support you as a caregiver, such as peer and professional support and organizations that help with respite. Nothing is more important than investing in and preserving your own mind.

ORGANIZATIONS

Alzheimer's Association
Helpline: 800-272-3900

Perhaps Alzheimer's Association's most import resource is the helpline, which is available 24/7. The helpline is staffed by master's-level mental health workers who are very well versed in dementia disorders. They are there for crisis intervention and emotional support, and they provide information, referrals, and guidance. Or, if are feeling alone and overwhelmed and simply need to talk, you can find a compassionate and knowledgeable person to speak to.

I Have Alzheimer's

alz.org/IHaveAlz
An online resource, created with input from individuals with Alzheimer's and other dementias, that offers information and strategies to help those living in the early stage of the disease lead their best lives for as long as possible.

Alzheimer's and Dementia Caregiver Center

alz.org/care
A resource for caregivers, family, and friends that provides reliable information and access to helpful online tools, including ALZConnected (alzconnected.org), an online community for people with dementia, caregivers, family, and friends, and Alzheimer's Navigator (alz.org/alzheimersnavigator), an innovative tool for creating a customized plan of action for life with Alz-

heimer's. The Navigator is a great resource if you don't know what your action plan should be and what you should prioritize. It asks you a few questions and, based on your responses, suggests different topics, like understanding the disease, home safety, financial planning, caregiver support, and so forth.

Community Resource Finder

alz.org/CRF
A tool for finding local resources and programs, like a support group or medical services.

Green-Field Library

alz.org/library
The nation's largest library dedicated to Alzheimer's disease, with material accessible virtually.

Early Stage Programs

alz.org/nca/helping_you/early_stage_programs
Resources for people living with Alzheimer's in its early stage.

Alzheimer's Foundation of America

alzfdn.org
This organization has a helpline (866-232-8484) that can help you with any practical questions, or if you simply need someone to talk to. They also provide support, services, and education to individuals, families, and caregivers affected by dementia disorders.

ALZHEIMER'S DISEASE INTERNATIONAL

alzint.org

A great resource if you want listings of Alzheimer's organizations and resources around the world. It also provides manuals, fact sheets, guidance for care plans, and up-to-date research and breakthroughs from researchers and dementia experts around the world.

HILARITY FOR CHARITY

wearehfc.org

One of my personal favorites, this organization has many resources, but it is well-known for respite grants, which are a huge sanity preserver for caregivers. And it has a variety of support groups, led by mental health care professionals who have expertise in dementia disorders. Many of these are for specific groups; there are young adult groups, long-distance groups, bereavement groups, and African American groups. The organization also hosts webinars and talks about subjects that affect dementia caregivers.

SAGE

sageusa.org

An organization that advocates for LGBTQ seniors, SAGE has information and resources and provides connection and wellness for the senior LGBTQ community. There are LGBTQ dementia caregiver support groups and trained professionals who can address issues of aging.

THE ASSOCIATION FOR FRONTOTEMPORAL DEGENERATION

theaftd.org

This organization specifically addresses the needs of families affected by frontotemporal degeneration (FTD), a dementia disorder that typical affects younger people and is more likely to get misdiagnosed. It is a particularly challenging dementia disorder, in part because it associated with inappropriate behavior due to personality changes and impairment to executive function. This organization helps provide information, support, and caregiving groups. It also has support for kids and teens. The helpline number is 1-866-507-7222.

THE LEWY BODY DEMENTIA ASSOCIATION

lbda.org

LBD is the second most common type of progressive dementia after Alzheimer's disease but is widely underdiagnosed. It shares a lot with Alzheimer's (and often individuals with LBD have Alzheimer's as well), but along with cognition it affects movement. This organization provides education, resources, and support, including LBD support groups. The helpline, also called the Lewy line, is 800-539-9767.

HELPFUL WEBSITES

ALZHEIMER'S STORE

alzstore.com

Sells gadgets such as simple universal remotes, automatic medication dispensers, easy-to-use phones and clocks, engaging games and fidget toys, etc.

ELDER CARE HELP

eldercare.acl.gov

This website allows you to enter your zip code to find local elder care agencies.

NATIONAL ACADEMY OF ELDER LAW ATTORNEYS

naela.org/findalawyer

A database for finding lawyers who specialize in elder law issues.

AMERICAN ASSOCIATION FOR GERIATRIC PSYCHIATRY

aagponline.org

A resource for finding psychiatric help (click "Find a Geriatric Psychiatrist" on the website). If you enter a specific city or town or zip code, the search engine will search only that location. To find someone nearby, try entering the state and leaving the city blank.

ROON

roon.com/dementia/home

An incredible platform, with curated videos answering questions from a wide variety of professional backgrounds as well as caregivers and people living with dementia. This can be a great tool because using a simple search engine like Google can lead to an overwhelming amount of information that has not been vetted.

Teepa Snow's Positive Approach to Care

teepasnow.com

Teepa Snow is renowned for her blunt and person-centered approach to communicating with people living with dementia (PLWD). On her website, you can learn about the disease, listen to her podcast, and take courses to improve your communication skills with PLWD. Many have found Snow's approach invaluable. Of course, no individual approach is going to work for everyone, and no single teacher can fit everyone's learning style. To get a sense of Teepa Snow's approach, you can always look at a few videos and see if it's a good fit for you.

Aging Life Care Association

aginglifecare.org

One of the organizations that has created a certification (although there's not a single gold-standard one) for geriatric care managers. This link goes to their database so you can search for someone in your area: aginglifecare.org/Shared_Content/ALCA_Directory/ALCA_Find_an_Expert.aspx?hkey=6c3ced7c-b5f0-4d27-9d30-37734ab6cf49

Psychology Today

psychologytoday.com

I have recommended this to my own clients looking for a therapist. You can search by location, insurance, approach, and mental health category. This can help you find a therapist who understands dementia disorder, or any other issue you are dealing with.

BEING PATIENT

beingpatient.com

A wonderful resource for caregivers and people living with dementia who want up-to-date brain research and dementia-related news from healthcare providers, scientists, researchers, and pharmaceutical and biotech innovators. In addition, the website offers stories from caregivers and patients, along with advice, guidance, and conversation with experts in the field.

DEMENTIA ACTION ALLIANCE

daanow.org

Online discussion groups, podcasts, and newsletters, as well as opportunities for connection for people living with dementia and their caregivers.

DEMENTIA SPRING

dementiaspring.org

Brings together the artistic and dementia communities to celebrate the impact that the visual and performing arts can have on the lives of those with dementia, their families, and caregivers.

LORENZO'S HOUSE

lorenzoshouse.org

Addresses the needs of those living with younger-onset dementia (sixty-five and younger) by providing education, respite grants, and support for the afflicted and their families.

ONLINE GUIDES

FAMILY CARE GUIDE

alz.org/media/manh/documents/alzheimer_s-family-care-guide
-(fcg).pdf

This manual comes from the Alzheimer's Association and provides a basic but thorough breakdown of the disease. It includes advice on dealing with challenging behaviors, navigating stressful situations like safety risks, addressing daily living needs of the PLWD, and addressing your own needs throughout. There is also general guidance on legal, financial, and medical steps that caregivers should take. This manual is great for beginners, to get a sense of where your priorities lie and to take it one step at a time.

NAVIGATING ALZHEIMER'S AND RELATED DEMENTIAS

umc.edu/mindcenter/files/Navigating-Alzheimers-Resource-
Guide_DIGITAL.pdf

Basic, easy to understand, and can help you build a road map for managing difficult behavior, safety concerns, and medications and for planning ahead.

DEMENTIA AUSTRALIA

dementia.org.au

One of the rare websites where you can find resources, guidance, education and advice in many different languages.

AARP

aarp.org/caregiving

AARP provides caregiving information on care at home, nursing homes, long-term care, life balance, and many other essential topics. It also has other resources and information, as well as stories from caregivers.

BOOKS

Nancy L. Mace and Peter V. Rabins, *The 36-Hour Day*
This has been a long-standing gold standard in dementia literature and has a lot of practical, hands-on advice to guide the caregiver. It can be overwhelming to realize how much you need to do as a caregiver. It's impossible to do everything all at once, so remember to pace yourself.

Gail Weatherill, *The Caregiver's Guide to Dementia*
This book explains the various kinds of dementias, provides caregiver wellness and mindfulness exercises, and lists practical resources, from financial planning to tips on safety, along with helpful questions for healthcare professionals, lawyers, accountants, therapists, and friends.

Pauline Boss, *Ambiguous Loss*
This is a seminal book in dementia literature. Pauline Boss introduces a key concept, "ambiguous loss," which helps frame the particular struggle of caregivers mourning someone who is still alive. Many caregivers I know found this work incredibly validating and supportive.

Renee Phillippi, *Dementia for Caregivers*
The author really focuses on stressful and challenging symptoms like delusions, aggression, issues around eating, and more. She provides practical, empathic approaches that can be tremendously helpful for a lot of families.

Oliver James, *Contented Dementia*
While the title might sound like a long shot for many caregivers, this book provides excellent tips for how to help a PLWD increase their quality of life. The author concentrates on the PLWD's capacity rather than deficits while preserving their sense of self and dignity. The guidance on how to approach and communicate with PLWD is woven together with anecdotal stories, making the advice easy to understand. Many caregivers learn how even small changes make a big difference.

Tia Powell, *Dementia Reimagined*
A favorite for many dementia professionals. It is not a guide, but it has given hope to a lot of caregivers and professionals. The beginning is much more historical/medical (interesting, although not directly applicable for most caregivers), but the second half helps guide families in thinking about dementia care, ethics, and existential questions. It does not solve practical concerns, but it can expand your thinking about dementia, which many find quite uplifting.

Olivia Ames Hoblitzelle, *Ten Thousand Joys and Ten Thousand Sorrows*
So many of my colleagues and friends in the field love this book. It balances the highs and lows of caregiving and gently reveals the emotional toll of the disease while also helping the reader find more peace and acceptance. If you are looking for something hopeful but also grounded, this might be the right book. Each chapter ends with reflections and suggestions that can provide readers something tangible to process and work on.

Thomas F. Harrison and Brent P. Forester, *The Complete Family Guide to Dementia*
This book addresses some of emotional aspects of the caregiver and includes practical tips. Reading it is like listening to a mentor who's been there gently walking you through. Although it's primarily addressed to caregivers who are adult children, it's still applicable to spouses.

Joanne Koenig Coste, *Learning to Speak Alzheimer's*
This is a book that is very gentle and compassionate toward PLWD and helps caregivers learn to live in the patient's reality. There are excellent communication tips throughout, but I do feel that it demands a lot of time and patience from caregivers, so please show yourself compassion as you go through it.

Arthur Kleinman, *The Soul of Care*
Kleinman is a physician who became a family caregiver. Despite his medical background, he approaches his experience

with humility and describes his caregiving with all the panic, wonder, tenderness, and humanity of any family caregiver who is overwhelmed by the emotional upheaval this disease creates.

Sandeep Jauhar, *My Father's Brain*
A personal favorite. Dr. Jauhar has written several bestselling books, and his latest is a memoir of caring for his father with Alzheimer's. It is beautifully written and refreshingly honest about the emotional toll of caregiving, the effect on the family as whole when coping with this illness, the ethical issues that come up, and the struggle to accept the illness and its demands.

Roberta Satow, *Doing the Right Thing: Taking Care of Your Elderly Parents Even If They Didn't Take Care of You*
Taking care of your parents is not easy, especially if a parent has been neglectful, unkind, or even abusive but this book offers a compassionate, validating look into adult children who are in this position. While the author does not give explicit guidance, she does emphasize the importance of self-care, boundaries, and being mindful of one's own feelings. For many, reading this book is like attending a support group in which one simply feels less alone. As with all support groups, I suggest that you take what resonates and leave the rest.

Notes

Preface

xxi   **"romantic science":** Luria had actually encouraged Sacks to continue writing case histories. Oliver Sacks, *The Man Who Mistook His Wife for a Hat and Other Clinical Tales* (Simon & Schuster, 1998), 5–6.

xxii   **"neurology's favorite word":** Sacks, *Man Who Mistook His Wife,* 3–6.

xxii   **leaning on our "cognitive reserve":** "Cognitive reserve" is a complex concept and usually refers to different kinds of resilience. Generally, it is a term that describes the difference between degree of brain damage and the outward manifestations of pathology. There are several models that account for a large discrepancy. One is the "brain reserve" model: Some people have a larger brain, with more neurons and synapses, which allows the brain to withstand pathology better. The way I use "cognitive reserve" is in keeping with the "active" model, which refers to the brain's ability to compensate for pathology by using alternative brain networks to function. Yaakov Stern et al., "Brain Reserve, Cognitive Reserve, Compensation, and Maintenance: Operationalization, Validity, and Mechanisms of Cognitive Resilience," *Neurobiology of Aging* 83 (2019): 124–29. For a review of lifestyle factors that can account for cognitive reserve, see Suhang Song, Yaakov Stern, and Yian Gu, "Modifiable Lifestyle Factors and Cognitive Reserve: A Systematic Review of Current Evidence," *Ageing Research Reviews* 74 (2022): 101551.

xxiii   **"a long-married couple":** Sacks was specifically referring to Tourette syndrome, but I believe this characterization also applies to dementia disorders. Oliver Sacks, *An Anthropologist on Mars: Seven Paradoxical Tales* (Vintage, 1995), 77.

xxiii   **"the preservation of the self":** Sacks, *Anthropologist on Mars*, xi.

xxv   **"charming, intelligent, memoryless":** Sacks, *Man Who Mistook His Wife,* 23.

xxvi   **"continuing pressure of anomaly and contradiction":** Sacks, *Man Who Mistook His Wife,* 29.

xxvi   ***The Diagnostic and Statistical Manual:*** Joseph R. Simpson, "DSM-5 and Neurocognitive Disorders," *Journal of the American Academy of Psychiatry and the Law Online* 42.2 (2014): 159–64.

xxvii   **More than fifty-five million people:** Joon-Ho Shin, "Dementia Epidemiology Fact Sheet 2022," *Annals of Rehabilitation Medicine* 46.2 (2022): 53.

xxvii   **some 6.5 million people:** Joseph Gaugler et al., "2022 Alzheimer's Disease Facts and Figures," *Alzheimer's and Dementia* 18.4 (2022): 700–789.

xxvii   **physical and psychological cost:** Henry Brodaty and Marika Donkin, "Family Caregivers of People with Dementia," *Dialogues in Clinical Neuroscience* 11.2 (2022): 217–28.

xxxi   **a woman with autism:** Sacks, *Anthropologist on Mars,* 244–96.

xxxii   **"heroes, victims, martyrs, warriors":** Sacks, *Man Who Mistook His Wife,* ix.

1   Borges in the Bronx

3   **a young man saddles his horse:** Jorge Luis Borges, "Funes the Memorious" (1962).

4   **"every leaf on every tree":** Ibid., 153.

4   **"I have more memories in myself alone":** Ibid., 152.

4   **"more ancient than Egypt":** Ibid., 154.

9   **In *The Seven Sins of Memory:*** Daniel L. Schacter, *The Seven Sins of Memory: How the Mind Forgets and Remembers* (Houghton Mifflin, 2002).

10   **to impose order on the environment:** Schacter is referencing the work of Gerald Edelman. Gerald Edelman, *Bright Air, Brilliant Fire* (Basic Books, 1992). Daniel L. Schacter, *Searching for Memory: The Brain, the Mind, and the Past* (Basic Books, 1996), 52.

10   **shining a spotlight on the past:** Schacter, *Searching for Memory,* 71.

10   **biochemical changes known as "engrams":** For a current

overview of engrams, see Sheena A. Josselyn and Susumu
Tonegawa, "Memory Engrams: Recalling the Past and Imagining the Future," *Science* 367.6473 (2020): eaaw4325.

10   **"one-to-one correspondence":** Ibid.

10–11 **"is not simply an activated engram":** Schacter, *Searching for
       Memory,* 71.

11   **The "personality knowledge" that forms our self-image:**
       Perrine Ruby et al., "Perspective Taking to Assess Self-
       Personality: What's Modified in Alzheimer's Disease?" *Neuro-
       biology of Aging* 30.10 (2009): 1637–51.

12   **memory's "egocentric bias":** In the chapter titled "The Sin of
       Bias," Schacter emphasizes the pervasive role "the self" plays on
       encoding and retrieving memory. The self is not a "neutral
       observer of the world," since it remembers past events in a
       "self-enhancing light." *Searching for Memory,* 150–53. For an
       example of egocentric bias at work, see Michael Ross and Fiore
       Sicoly, "Egocentric Biases in Availability and Attribution,"
       Journal of Personality and Social Psychology 37.3 (1979): 322.
       For a review of the self's overwhelming influence on memory,
       see Anthony G. Greenwald, "The Totalitarian Ego," *American
       Psychologist* 35.7 (1980): 603–18; Cynthia S. Symons and Blair
       T. Johnson, "The Self-Reference Effect in Memory: A Meta-
       analysis," *Psychological Bulletin* 121.3 (1997): 371; and Martin
       A. Conway, "Memory and the Self," *Journal of Memory and
       Language* 53.4 (2005): 594–628. For a discussion of how
       memory is self-protecting, see Constantine Sedikides and
       Jeffrey D. Green, "Memory as a Self-Protective Mechanism,"
       Social and Personality Psychology Compass 3.6 (2009): 1055–68.

13   **"continuity, a narrative continuity":** Oliver Sacks, "The
       Abyss: Music and Amnesia," *New Yorker* 24 (2007): 100–112.

13   **memory is biased toward preexisting knowledge:** Garvin
       Brod, Markus Werkle-Bergner, and Yee Lee Shing, "The
       Influence of Prior Knowledge on Memory: a Developmental
       Cognitive Neuroscience Perspective," *Frontiers in Behavioral
       Neuroscience* 7 (2013): 139.

17   **There is *explicit* memory:** For a review of explicit and
       implicit memory, see Daniel L. Schacter, C.-Y. Peter Chiu, and
       Kevin N. Ochsner, "Implicit Memory: A Selective Review,"
       Annual Review of Neuroscience 16.1 (1993): 159–82. For
       current research on implicit memory, see Daniel L. Schacter,
       "Implicit Memory, Constructive Memory, and Imagining the
       Future: A Career Perspective," *Perspectives on Psychological
       Science* 14.2 (2019): 256–72.

17   **When amnesia patients in one experiment:** Alan J. Parkin,
       "Residual Learning Capability in Organic Amnesia," *Cortex*
       18.3 (1982): 417–40. Indeed, not just fear but feelings of

happiness and sadness can persist. Justin S. Feinstein, Melissa C. Duff, and Daniel Tranel, "Sustained Experience of Emotion After Loss of Memory in Patients with Amnesia," *Proceedings of the National Academy of Sciences* 107.17 (2010): 7674–79.

18   **Our mind abhors ambiguity:** Vilayanur S. Ramachandran and Diane Rogers-Ramachandran, "Hidden in Plain Sight," *Scientific American Mind* 16.4 (2005): 16–18. Most of our aversion to ambiguity has been studied as it relates to the visual system. But as Daniel Kahneman explains in his seminal book *Thinking, Fast and Slow,* our brain naturally suppresses ambiguity and creates the feeling of cohesion because it's easier on our brain. Daniel Kahneman, *Thinking, Fast and Slow* (Farrar, Straus and Giroux, 2013), 79–83.

19   **"a dog at three-fourteen":** Borges, "Funes," 153.

2   "The Weak Child"

22   "**monstrous verminous bug**": Franz Kafka, *The Metamorphosis* (Schocken Books, 1948).

28   **what the British psychologist John Bowlby calls a "secure base":** John Bowlby, "Attachment and Loss: Retrospect and Prospect," *American Journal of Orthopsychiatry* 52.4 (1982): 664.

28   **tend to develop defensive coping strategies:** Mary D. Salter Ainsworth, "Attachment as Related to Mother-Infant Interaction," in Jay S. Rosenblatt et al., *Advances in the Study of Behavior,* vol. 9 (Academic Press, 1979), 1–51.

28–29   **affect how we move through the world:** Bowlby posited that the attachment systems affect us across our lifespan from "cradle to grave." Bowlby, "Attachment and Loss." A good overview of how the attachment systems inform many aspects of ourselves and others and how we deal with stress can be found in Mario Mikulincer and Phillip R. Shaver, "The Attachment Behavioral System in Adulthood: Activation, Psychodynamics, and Interpersonal Processes," in M. P. Zanna, ed., *Advances in Experimental Social Psychology,* vol. 35 (New York: Academic Press, 2003), 53–152.

31   **"cognitive revolution":** Howard Gardner, *The Mind's New Science: A History of the Cognitive Revolution* (Basic Books, 1987).

31   **"the tip of the iceberg":** Sigmund Freud, "The Unconscious" (1915), in *Standard Edition of the Complete Psychological Works,* vol. 14 (London: Hogarth, 1959): 166–201.

31   **hummed along independently of consciousness:** John F. Kihlstrom, "The Cognitive Unconscious," *Science* 237.4821 (1987): 1445–52.

31   **"part of the architecture of the brain":** Timothy D. Wilson,
        Strangers to Ourselves: Discovering the Adaptive Unconscious
        (Cambridge, Mass.: Harvard University Press, 2002).

32   **This "adaptive unconscious," a term first coined:** Daniel
        M. Wegner, "Précis of the Illusion of Conscious Will," *Behavioral and Brain Sciences* 27.5 (2004): 649–59.

32   **referred to as "zombie subsystems":** Christof Koch and
        Francis Crick, "The Zombie Within," *Nature* 411.6840 (2001):
        893.

32   **unconscious processes can also involve:** Expertise, skill,
        habits, pursuit of goals, and many other sophisticated cognitive
        processes are part of the unconscious repertoire and do not
        require the mental effort of conscious processes. John A. Bargh
        and Melissa J. Ferguson, "Beyond Behaviorism: On the
        Automaticity of Higher Mental Processes," *Psychological
        Bulletin* 126.6 (2000): 925; John A. Bargh et al., "The Automated Will: Nonconscious Activation and Pursuit of Behavioral
        Goals," *Journal of Personality and Social Psychology* 81.6 (2001):
        1014; John A. Bargh and Erin L. Williams, "The Automaticity
        of Social Life," *Current Directions in Psychological Science* 15.1
        (2006): 1–4.

32–33   **we generally believe that judgment, thinking, and
        character are all guided:** We tend to feel (and thus overestimate) conscious will when we act and make decisions. Wegner,
        "Précis of the Illusion of Conscious Will"; Ruud Custers and
        Henk Aarts, "The Unconscious Will: How the Pursuit of Goals
        Operates Outside of Conscious Awareness," *Science* 329.5987
        (2010): 47–50; Roy F. Baumeister, E. J. Masicampo, and
        Kathleen D. Vohs, "Do Conscious Thoughts Cause Behavior?"
        Annual Review of Psychology 62 (2011): 331–61; John A. Bargh
        and Ezequiel Morsella, "The Unconscious Mind," *Perspectives
        on Psychological Science* 3.1 (2008): 73–79. It makes sense that
        we underestimate our automatic processes and by extension
        overestimate consciousness, since, as Wilson points out, our
        lack of awareness is one of the defining features of the unconscious. Wilson, *Strangers to Ourselves*, 5. This subject is
        addressed more fully in chapter 5.

33   **derive from unconscious processes:** Wilson, *Strangers to
        Ourselves*, 22.

34   **sledding analogy:** Norman Doidge, *The Brain That Changes
        Itself: Stories of Personal Triumph from the Frontiers of Brain
        Science* (New York: Penguin, 2007): 209.

35   **attachment behaviors that emerge in response to stress:**
        Bowlby believed that attachment systems are especially evident
        in times of ill health and loss. John Bowlby, "The Bowlby-
        Ainsworth Attachment Theory," *Behavioral and Brain Sciences*

2.4 (1979): 637–38. Researchers have supported Bowlby's assertion, finding that attachment systems become more activated with aging, and with dementia disorders in particular. C. J. Browne and E. Shlosberg, "Attachment Theory, Ageing and Dementia: A Review of the Literature," *Aging and Mental Health* 10.2 (2006): 134–42. Indeed, in the face of loss, distress, or illness, a person will tend to seek an "attachment figure." Giacomo d'Elia, "Attachment: A Biological Basis for the Therapeutic Relationship?" *Nordic Journal of Psychiatry* 55.5 (2001): 329–36. Since the "attachment figure" for dementia patients is usually the caregiver, it's no wonder that they are the recipients of the patient's repetitive behavior, such as shadowing, clinging, constant calling out for them, and general fixations on objects and places that represent safety.

35   **can create an internal climate:** The dementia researcher Bère Miesen proposes that people with dementia disorders can still respond to their illness even after their "illness insight" has disappeared, because the disease creates constant stress related to separation, loss, powerlessness, and displacement. This is the source of what he found to be a dementia patient's "parent fixation" in nursing homes. Bère M. L. Miesen, "Alzheimer's Disease, the Phenomenon of Parent Fixation and Bowlby's Attachment Theory," *International Journal of Geriatric Psychiatry* 8.2 (1993): 147–53; Bère Miesen, *Dementia in Close-up: Understanding and Caring for People with Dementia* (Routledge, 1999). Other researchers have had similar findings; see, for example, Hannah Osborne, Graham Stokes, and Jane Simpson, "A Psychosocial Model of Parent Fixation in People with Dementia: The Role of Personality and Attachment," *Aging and Mental Health* 14.8 (2010): 928–37.

35   **Alzheimer's didn't suddenly change this:** Although very little research has been done on this subject, it appears that premorbid attachment styles continue to affect how patients cope with Alzheimer's and how symptoms manifest. Carol Magai and Stewart I. Cohen, "Attachment Style and Emotion Regulation in Dementia Patients and Their Relation to Caregiver Burden," *Journals of Gerontology. Series B: Psychological Sciences and Social Sciences* 53.3 (1998): 147–54.

37   **a caregiver's own attachment system can't help but get triggered:** Unfortunately, not much work has been done on how attachment affects the dyad. Caregivers' attachment is also triggered by dementia disorders. Reidun Ingebretsen and Per Erik Solem, "Spouses of Persons with Dementia: Attachment, Loss and Coping," *Norsk Epidemiologi* 8.2 (1998).

38   **switch over from unconscious to conscious responses:**
Automatic and controlled processes tend to differ. Automatic
(our brain's preferred state) is efficient, effortless, rigid, and
difficult to stop. Consciousness is effortful, flexible, and
cognitively more depleting. Robert S. Wyer, Jr., *The Automaticity of Everyday Life: Advances in Social Cognition,* vol. X
(Psychology Press, 2014). For a handy guide to unconscious
versus conscious characteristics, see Wilson, *Strangers to
Ourselves,* 49.

38   **The brain's objective:** It is adaptive for our brain not to
concern itself with perfect reason but to settle for "good
enough." This is the idea behind the research done on
"bounded rationality," which reveals that our brain risks
making mistakes and leading us astray as a trade-off for
ease and efficiency. Gerd Gigerenzer and Reinhard Selten,
eds., *Bounded Rationality: The Adaptive Toolbox* (MIT Press,
2002).

38   **but to conserve energy:** Our brain has been characterized as
"lazy," a "cognitive miser," generally preferring to be "fast and
frugal" and tending to pursue the line of "least mental effort,"
favoring habit over difficult change. W. J. McGuire, "The
Nature of Attitudes and Attitude Change," in Elliot Aronson
and Gardner Lindzey, eds., *The Handbook of Social Psychology,*
2nd ed., vol. 3 (Addison-Wesley, 1969), 136–314; Shelley E.
Taylor, "The Interface of Cognitive and Social Psychology,"
Cognition, Social Behavior, and the Environment 1 (1981):
189–211; Gerd Gigerenzer and Daniel G. Goldstein, "Reasoning the Fast and Frugal Way: Models of Bounded Rationality,"
Psychological Review 103.4 (1996): 650; Michael Ballé, "La loi
du moindre effort mental: Les représentations mentales,"
Sciences humaines (Auxerre) 128 (2002): 36–39; A. David
Redish, *The Mind Within the Brain: How We Make Decisions
and How Those Decisions Go Wrong* (Oxford University Press,
2013); Wouter Kool et al., "Decision Making and the Avoidance
of Cognitive Demand," *Journal of Experimental Psychology:
General* 139.4 (2010): 665.

38   **pricey conscious activities:** One of the defining characteristics of conscious processes is that they are inherently effortful
and consequently cost the brain more energy. Jan–Åke Nilsson,
"Metabolic Consequences of Hard Work," *Proceedings of the
Royal Society of London. Series B: Biological Sciences* 269.1501
(2002): 1735–39.

38   **our brains become especially frugal:** We will see in chapter
5 why our mind quickly turns to efficient unconscious processes when it is taxed or depleted.

3 Dementia Blindness

40   **The Müller-Lyer illusion:** Franz Carl Müller-Lyer, *Formen der Ehe, der Familie und der Verwandtschaft,* vol. 3 (J. F. Lehmann, 1911).

41   **In *Thinking, Fast and Slow:*** Daniel Kahneman, *Thinking, Fast and Slow* (Farrar, Straus and Giroux, 2013), 19–30.

43   **the real blind spot:** Gordon L. Walls, "The Filling-In Process," *Optometry and Vision Science* 31.7 (1954): 329–41; Vilayanur S. Ramachandran, "Blind Spots," *Scientific American* 266.5 (1992): 86–91. For a review of when our perceptual system fills in and when it doesn't, see Lothar Spillmann et al., "Perceptual Filling-In from the Edge of the Blind Spot," *Vision Research* 46.25 (2006): 4252–57.

44   **the Hollow-Face illusion:** See Richard L. Gregory, "The Confounded Eye," *Illusion in Nature and Art* (1973), 49–96.

45   **the cognitive scientist Andy Clark:** Specifically, the glitches or mistakes that we make are a trade-off for seeing a world that's more stable, less ambiguous, and less noisy, which in turn allows us to navigate it with greater ease and efficiency. Andy Clark, *Surfing Uncertainty: Prediction, Action, and the Embodied Mind* (Oxford University Press, 2016), 51.

45   **direct access to the outside world:** We have a tendency to believe that our perceptions of the world reflect how it actually looks. As a result, we overestimate our accuracy and objectivity. This bias, called naïve realism, holds true for our visual perceptions as well as our day-to-day worldviews. Harvey S. Smallman and Mark John, "Naive Realism: Limits of Realism as a Display Principle," *Proceedings of the Human Factors and Ergonomics Society Annual Meeting* 49, no. 17 (2005); Andrew Ward, "Naive Realism in Everyday Life: Implications for Social Conflict," *Values and Knowledge* 103 (1996).

46   **is known as "bottom-up perception":** David Marr, *Vision: A Computational Investigation into the Human Representation and Processing of Visual Information* (San Francisco: W. H. Freeman, 1982).

46   **is referred to as "top-down processing":** This idea can be traced back to Helmholtz's theory of unconscious inference. Hermann von Helmholtz, *Handbuch der Physiologischen Optik: Mit 213 in den Text Eingedruckten Holzschnitten und 11 Tafeln,* vol. 9 (Voss, 1867). Current examples of active or "top-down" argument can be found in Patricia S. Churchland, Vilayanur S. Ramachandran, and Terrence J. Sejnowski, "A Critique of Pure Vision," in *Large-Scale Neuronal Theories of the Brain,* ed. Christof Koch and Joel L. David (MIT Press, 1993); Andy Clark, "Whatever Next? Predictive Brains, Situated Agents, and

the Future of Cognitive Science," *Behavioral and Brain Sciences* 36.3 (2013): 181–204; Andy Clark, "Perceiving as Predicting," *Perception and Its Modalities* (2014): 23–43.

46 **Without an internal model of the world:** For a review of the usefulness of the internal model, see Tai Sing Lee, "The Visual System's Internal Model of the World," *Proceedings of the IEEE* 103.8 (2015): 1359–78.

47 **"a rich background of prior knowledge":** Clark, *Surfing Uncertainty,* 225.

47 **"narrative fallacies":** Nassim Nicholas Taleb, *The Black Swan: The Impact of the Highly Improbable* (Random House, 2007), 63–84.

52 **B. F. Skinner placed hungry pigeons in a box:** Burrhus Frederic Skinner, "'Superstition' in the Pigeon," *Journal of Experimental Psychology* 38.2 (1948): 168.

52 **the source of superstition, magical thinking, and ritualistic behavior:** Cognitive psychologists have supported Skinner's research on superstition as a by-product of accidental learning, which requires making associations. Jan Beck and Wolfgang Forstmeier, "Superstition and Belief as Inevitable By-Products of an Adaptive Learning Strategy," *Human Nature* 18.1 (2007): 35–46.

52 **gave rewards to mice at random:** B. F. Skinner, "The Experimental Analysis of Behavior," *American Scientist* 45.4 (1957): 343–71.

53 **The same might be said of human beings:** Gregory J. Madden, Eric E. Ewan, and Carla H. Lagorio, "Toward an Animal Model of Gambling: Delay Discounting and the Allure of Unpredictable Outcomes," *Journal of Gambling Studies* 23.1 (2007): 63–83.

53 **Our normal, selective memory fastens:** Daniel L. Schacter, "The Seven Sins of Memory: Insights from Psychology and Cognitive Neuroscience," *American Psychologist* 54.3 (1999): 182.

53 **As the science writer Michael Shermer explains:** *The Believing Brain: From Ghosts and Gods to Politics and Conspiracies—How We Construct Beliefs and Reinforce Them as Truths* (New York: St. Martin's Griffin, 2012).

53 **It's safer, after all, to believe:** For a discussion of why we feel it is safer to assume cause and effect between two events, see Kevin R. Foster and Hanna Kokko, "The Evolution of Superstitious and Superstition-like Behaviour," *Proceedings of the Royal Society of London. Series B: Biological Sciences* 276.1654 (2009): 31–37.

53 **we sometimes make false, even bizarre connections:** Shermer, *Believing Brain,* 62.

53 **more likely to see patterns where none exist:** Jennifer A. Whitson and Adam D. Galinsky, "Lacking Control Increases Illusory Pattern Perception," *Science* 322.5898 (2008): 115–17.

54 **cognitive illusions can be just as convincing:** Cognitive illusions are just as hard to overcome because, like visual illusions, they run automatically. It is hard to "turn them off" because that requires the vigilance and constant questioning that our adaptively lazy brain tends to avoid. Kahneman, *Thinking, Fast and Slow,* 27–28.

4   Chekhov and the Left-Brain Interpreter

60 **has termed the "left-brain interpreter":** Michael S. Gazzaniga and Joseph E. LeDoux, "The Split Brain and the Integrated Mind," in *The Integrated Mind* (Springer, 1978), 1–7; Michael S. Gazzaniga, "Organization of the Human Brain," *Science* 245.4921 (1989): 947–52; Michael S. Gazzaniga, "Cerebral Specialization and Interhemispheric Communication: Does the Corpus Callosum Enable the Human Condition?" *Brain* 123.7 (2000): 1293–1326.

60 **if "hijacked" by bad information:** Michael Gazzaniga, *Who's in Charge? Free Will and the Science of the Brain* (Ecco, 2012), 94–95.

61 **Capgras syndrome:** William Hirstein and Vilayanur S. Ramachandran, "Capgras Syndrome: A Novel Probe for Understanding the Neural Representation of the Identity and Familiarity of Persons," *Proceedings of the Royal Society of London. Series B: Biological Sciences* 264.1380 (1997): 437–44.

61 **the person does not *feel* like Mom:** John M. Doran, "The Capgras Syndrome: Neurological/Neuropsychological Perspec- tives," *Neuropsychology* 4.1 (1990): 29.

62 **administered epinephrine:** Stanley Schachter and Jerome Singer, "Cognitive, Social, and Physiological Determinants of Emotional State," *Psychological Review* 69.5 (1962): 379.

65 **is not . . . an "all or nothing affair":** Patricia Churchland, *Brain-wise: Studies in Neurophilosophy* (MIT Press, 2002), 64.

66 **Paul Bloom refers to as the "essential self":** The notion of the "true self" is an extension of the essentialism that is found in our early development. Paul Bloom, "Précis of How Children Learn the Meanings of Words," *Behavioral and Brain Sciences* 24.6 (2001): 1095–1103; Paul Bloom, "Water as an Artifact Kind," in *Creations of the Mind: Theories of Artifacts and Their Representation* (Oxford University Press: 2007), 150–56.

66 **a permanent "deep-down self":** Nina Strohminger, Joshua Knobe, and George Newman, "The True Self: A Psychological Concept Distinct from the Self," *Perspectives on Psychological*

Science 12.4 (2017): 551–60; Andrew G. Christy, Rebecca J. Schlegel, and Andrei Cimpian, "Why Do People Believe in a 'True Self'? The Role of Essentialist Reasoning About Personal Identity and the Self," *Journal of Personality and Social Psychology* 117.2 (2019): 386.

66 **When experimental philosophers, interested:** Nina Strohminger and Shaun Nichols, "The Essential Moral Self," *Cognition* 131.1 (2014): 159–71.

67 **to associate the "good" qualities in people with their true selves:** George E. Newman, Paul Bloom, and Joshua Knobe, "Value Judgments and the True Self," *Personality and Social Psychology Bulletin* 40.2 (2014): 203–16; Strohminger, Knobe, and Newman, "The True Self"; Julian De Freitas et al., "Consistent Belief in a Good True Self in Misanthropes and Three Interdependent Cultures," *Cognitive Science* 42 (2018): 134–60.

71 **The "experiencing self" is, of course, transient:** Daniel Kahneman and Jason Riis, "Living, and Thinking About It: Two Perspectives on Life," *The Science of Well-Being* 1 (2005): 285–304.

71 **Chekhov's *Uncle Vanya*:** Eugene K. Bristow, ed., *Anton Chekhov's Plays* (W. W. Norton, 1977), 95.

5 The Insistent, Persistent CEO

80 **the intuition that we have volition and free will:** Gazzaniga, *Who's in Charge?* 44–73.

80 **comparing consciousness to the CEO of a big company:** David Eagleman, *Incognito: The Secret Lives of the Brain* (Vintage, 2012), 143.

80–81 **Benjamin Libet measured consciousness's role in behavior:** This seminal study spurred a great deal of debate. It should be noted that Libet did not believe his study showed there is no free will. He still contends that consciousness has "veto power." Benjamin Libet, Curtis A. Gleason, Elwood W. Wright, and Dennis K. Pearl, "Time of Conscious Intention to Act in Relation to Onset of Cerebral Activity (Readiness-Potential): The Unconscious Initiation of a Freely Voluntary Act," *Brain* 106 (1983): 623; Benjamin Libet, "Unconscious Cerebral Initiative and the Role of Conscious Will in Voluntary Action," *Behavioral and Brain Sciences* 8.4 (1985): 529–39; Benjamin Libet, "Do We Have Free Will?" *Journal of Consciousness Studies* 6.8–9 (1999): 47–57. There are many critiques of the Libet study. Some have argued that the study is too "superficial" or "insignificant" to reveal something as complex as the nature of free will. Others have challenged the validity of "readiness potential." For a review of criticism and support, see Eoin Travers, Maja Friedemann, and Patrick Haggard, "The Readiness Potential Reflects Expectation, Not Uncertainty, in the Timing of Action," *bioRxiv* (2020).

81 **"the mind's best trick":** Daniel M. Wegner, "The Mind's Best Trick: How We Experience Conscious Will," *Trends in Cognitive Sciences* 7.2 (2003): 65–69.

81 **In one well-known experiment:** David Eagleman, *The Brain: The Story of You* (Pantheon, 2015), 94–95; Joaquim Pereira Brasil-Neto et al., "Focal Transcranial Magnetic Stimulation and Response Bias in a Forced-Choice Task," *Journal of Neurology, Neurosurgery and Psychiatry* 55.10 (1992): 964–66.

82 **When judges, for instance, justify their verdicts:** On racial biases, see Jeffrey J. Rachlinski et al., "Does Unconscious Racial Bias Affect Trial Judges?" *Notre Dame Law Review* 84 (2008): 1195, and David Arnold, Will Dobbie, and Crystal S. Yang, "Racial Bias in Bail Decisions," *Quarterly Journal of Economics* 133.4 (2018): 1885–1932. On general biases and heuristic mistakes, see Eyal Peer and Eyal Gamliel, "Heuristics and Biases in Judicial Decisions," *Court Review* 49 (2013): 114. On the effect of hunger pains on parole decisions, see Shai Danziger, Jonathan Levav, and Liora Avnaim-Pesso, "Extraneous Factors in Judicial Decisions," *Proceedings of the National Academy of Sciences* 108.17 (2011): 6889–92. On the effects of bad weather and last night's game on judicial decisions, see Daniel L. Chen, "This Morning's Breakfast, Last Night's Game: Detecting Extraneous Factors in Judging," IAST Working Papers 16-49, Institute for Advanced Study in Toulouse, 2016. It is important to note that there has been criticism of the "hungry judges study." See Andreas Glöckner, "The Irrational Hungry Judge Effect Revisited: Simulations Reveal That the Magnitude of the Effect Is Overestimated," *Judgment and Decision Making* 11.6 (2016): 601.

82 **consciousness plays a crucial role in mediating conflict:** Crick and Koch argue that consciousness exists to control the zombie systems. Francis Crick and Christof Koch, "Constraints on Cortical and Thalamic Projections: The No-Strong-Loops Hypothesis," *Nature* 391.6664 (1998): 245–50.

82 **we would have no cognitive flexibility:** Eagleman, *Incognito,* 142.

84 **of plural, localized consciousnesses:** Michael S. Gazzaniga, *The Consciousness Instinct: Unraveling the Mystery of How the Brain Makes the Mind* (Farrar, Straus and Giroux, 2018).

84 **If consciousness existed in only a single location:** Mark E. Nelson and James M. Bower, "Brain Maps and Parallel Computers," *Trends in Neurosciences* 13.10 (1990): 403–408.

86 **treating the mind and body as separate entities:** Paul Bloom, *Descartes' Baby: How the Science of Child Development Explains What Makes Us Human* (Basic Books, 2005).

86 **It's a default stance found across cultures:** Maciej Chudek et al., "Developmental and Cross-Cultural Evidence for Intuitive Dualism," *Psychological Science* 20 (2013): 1–19; Maira Roazzi, Melanie Nyhof, and Carl Johnson, "Mind, Soul and Spirit: Conceptions of Immaterial Identity in Different Cultures," *International Journal for the Psychology of Religion* 23.1 (2013): 75–86; H. Clark Barrett et al., "Intuitive Dualism and Afterlife Beliefs: A Cross-Cultural Study," *Cognitive Science* 45.6 (2021): e12992.

86 **"card-carrying dualists":** The social neuroscientist Matthew Lieberman explains that all of us are dualists because there is a neural chasm in the brain between how we think about minds and how we think about bodies. Matthew D. Lieberman, *Social: Why Our Brains Are Wired to Connect* (New York: Crown, 2014), 186.

87 **part of our cognitive architecture:** Different areas in the brain are implicated in reasoning about the physical world versus the mental world. Rebecca Saxe and Nancy Kanwisher, "People Thinking About Thinking People: The Role of the Temporo-Parietal Junction in 'Theory of Mind,'" in Gary G. Berntson and John T. Cacioppo, eds., *Social Neuroscience* (Psychology Press, 2013), 171–82. Studies in child development show that babies naturally think about physical objects and mental states differently. Valerie A. Kuhlmeier, Paul Bloom, and Karen Wynn, "Do 5-Month-Old Infants See Humans as Material Objects?" *Cognition* 94.1 (2004): 95–103; Maria Legerstee, "A Review of the Animate-Inanimate Distinction in Infancy: Implications for Models of Social and Cognitive Knowing," *Early Development and Parenting* 1.2 (1992): 59–67.

87 **"there's still a 'ghost in the machine'":** Gilbert Ryle, *The Concept of Mind* (Routledge, 2009).

88 **gets away from the dualism:** Even neuroscientists who decidedly reject the mind-body distinction still revert to using dualistic concepts and language in their writings. Liad Mudrik and Uri Maoz, "'Me and My Brain': Exposing Neuroscience's Closet Dualism," *Journal of Cognitive Neuroscience* 27.2 (2015): 211–21.

6 When Every Day Is Sunday

91 **religion, another "safe base":** God can also act as a noncorporal attachment figure. Aaron D. Cherniak et al., "Attachment Theory and Religion," *Current Opinion in Psychology* 40 (2021): 126–30.

93   **Human beings are "ultra-social" animals:** Michael
      Tomasello, "The Ultra-Social Animal," *European Journal of
      Social Psychology* 44.3 (2014): 187–94.

93   **this need for a mutually agreed-upon reality:** Gerald
      Echterhoff, E. Tory Higgins, and John M. Levine, "Shared
      Reality: Experiencing Commonality with Others' Inner States
      About the World," *Perspectives on Psychological Science* 4.5
      (2009): 496–521; Gerald Echterhoff and E. Tory Higgins,
      "Shared Reality: Construct and Mechanisms," *Current Opinion
      in Psychology* 23 (2018): iv–vii.

93   **we naturally overestimate the degree:** Humans have a
      tendency to use their knowledge, beliefs, and expertise as a
      proxy for what others feel and believe. This bias is believed to
      be a side effect of what psychologists call our natural "egocen-
      tricity" in perspective taking. One example of this is called
      "false consensus effect," which is a bias that leads us to think
      that others share our point of view more than they actually do.
      Lee Ross, David Greene, and Pamela House, "The 'False
      Consensus Effect': An Egocentric Bias in Social Perception
      and Attribution Processes," *Journal of Experimental Social
      Psychology* 13.3 (1977): 279–301; Boaz Keysar, Linda E.
      Ginzel, and Max H. Bazerman, "States of Affairs and States of
      Mind: The Effect of Knowledge of Beliefs," *Organizational
      Behavior and Human Decision Processes* 64.3 (1995): 283–93;
      Nicholas Epley et al., "Perspective Taking as Egocentric
      Anchoring and Adjustment," *Journal of Personality and Social
      Psychology* 87.3 (2004): 327; Nicholas Epley, Carey K.
      Morewedge, and Boaz Keysar, "Perspective Taking in Children
      and Adults: Equivalent Egocentrism but Differential Correc-
      tion," *Journal of Experimental Social Psychology* 40.6 (2004):
      760–68. There is also a bias called the "curse of knowledge,"
      which leads us to overestimate the degree to which people
      know about something we have learned or are experts in. Colin
      Camerer, George Loewenstein, and Martin Weber, "The Curse
      of Knowledge in Economic Settings: An Experimental Analy-
      sis," *Journal of Political Economy* 97.5 (1989): 1232–54; Susan
      A. J. Birch et al., "A 'Curse of Knowledge' in the Absence of
      Knowledge? People Misattribute Fluency When Judging How
      Common Knowledge Is Among Their Peers," *Cognition* 166
      (2017): 447–58. There is also the illusion of transparency,
      which leads us to overestimate how much people share in
      knowing about how we are feeling. Thomas Gilovich, Kenneth
      Savitsky, and Victoria Husted Medvec, "The Illusion of
      Transparency: Biased Assessments of Others' Ability to Read
      One's Emotional States," *Journal of Personality and Social
      Psychology* 75.2 (1998): 332.

94   **prefrontal cortex (PFC), where self-regulation takes place:** James A. Coan and John J. B. Allen, "Frontal EEG Asymmetry as a Moderator and Mediator of Emotion," *Biological Psychology* 67.1–2 (2004): 7–50; James A. Coan, John J. B. Allen, and Patrick E. McKnight, "A Capability Model of Individual Differences in Frontal EEG Asymmetry," *Biological Psychology* 72.2 (2006): 198–207. A meta-analysis shows the right and left ventrolateral prefrontal cortices as essential in emotion regulation. Nils Kohn et al., "Neural Network of Cognitive Emotion Regulation—an ALE Meta-analysis and MACM Analysis," *Neuroimage* 87 (2014): 345–55.

94   **two kinds of regulation strategies:** Automatic forms of regulation are associated with the ventromedial and medial orbital PFC. Mohammed R. Milad et al., "Thickness of Ventromedial Prefrontal Cortex in Humans Is Correlated with Extinction Memory," *Proceedings of the National Academy of Sciences* 102.30 (2005): 13; Gregory Quirk and Jennifer S. Beer, "Prefrontal Involvement in the Regulation of Emotion: Convergence of Rat and Human Studies," *Current Opinion in Neurobiology* 16.6 (2006): 723–27; Demetrio Sierra-Mercado, Jr., et al., "Inactivation of the Ventromedial Prefrontal Cortex Reduces Expression of Conditioned Fear and Impairs Subsequent Recall of Extinction," *European Journal of Neuroscience* 24.6 (2006): 1751–58.

94–95 **Self-regulation is effortful:** Effortful forms of regulation require more attention, working memory, and reappraisal associated with the lateral portion of the PFC. Kevin N. Ochsner et al., "Rethinking Feelings: An FMRI Study of the Cognitive Regulation of Emotion," *Journal of Cognitive Neuroscience* 14.8 (2002): 1215–29; Kevin N. Ochsner and James J. Gross, "The Cognitive Control of Emotion," *Trends in Cognitive Sciences* 9.5 (2005): 242–49. Feeling social support saves the brain from the metabolically costly job of effortful regulation in the PFC. It seems to happen on a subcortical level. Lane Beckes and James A. Coan, "Social Baseline Theory: The Role of Social Proximity in Emotion and Economy of Action," *Social and Personality Psychology Compass* 5.12 (2011): 976–88; Lane Beckes and David A. Sbarra, "Social Baseline Theory: State of the Science and New Directions," *Current Opinion in Psychology* 43 (2022): 36–41.

95   **we have evolved to co-regulate one another:** Dennis R. Proffitt, "Embodied Perception and the Economy of Action," *Perspectives on Psychological Science* 1.2 (2006): 110–22; James A. Coan and David A. Sbarra, "Social Baseline Theory: The Social Regulation of Risk and Effort," *Current Opinion in Psychology* 1 (2015): 87–91.

95   **as we would against ourselves:** Lane Beckes, James A.
        Coan, and Karen Hasselmo, "Familiarity Promotes the Blurring
        of Self and Other in the Neural Representation of Threat,"
        Social Cognitive and Affective Neuroscience 8.6 (2013): 670–77.

95   **what psychologists call *load sharing*:** James A. Coan,
        "Toward a Neuroscience of Attachment," in Jude Cassidy and
        Phillip R. Shaver, eds., *Handbook of Attachment: Theory,
        Research, and Clinical Applications,* 2nd ed. (New York:
        Guilford Press, 2008), 241–68.

95   **people in healthy and supportive relationships:** James A.
        Coan, Hillary S. Schaefer, and Richard J. Davidson, "Lending a
        Hand: Social Regulation of the Neural Response to Threat,"
        Psychological Science 17.12 (2006): 1032–39.

96   **Unfairness marks a loss of social connection:** Matthew D.
        Lieberman and Naomi I. Eisenberger, "Pains and Pleasures of
        Social Life," *Science* 323.5916 (2009): 890–91.

96   **Fairness . . . "tastes like chocolate":** The same regions that
        register loving chocolate (and other pleasures) love fairness,
        which also feels deeply rewarding. Lieberman, *Social,* 75.

97   **Loneliness shortens attention span:** John Cacioppo and
        William Patrick, *Loneliness: Human Nature and the Need for
        Social Connection* (W. W. Norton, 2009), 35–51.

97   **Self-control . . . is already a limited resource:** Limited
        because different types of willpower dip into the same energy
        source. Matthew T. Gailliot et al., "Self-control Relies on
        Glucose as a Limited Energy Source: Willpower Is More than a
        Metaphor," *Journal of Personality and Social Psychology* 92.2
        (2007): 325.

97   **dealing with someone's delusions:** Kahneman explains that
        we make more "intuitive errors" and have a harder time
        resisting temptation (from cigarettes to cookies) when we are in
        a state of ego depletion. Kahneman, *Thinking, Fast and Slow,*
        42–44. No wonder caregivers have a hard time overcoming all
        the intuitions that are required to deal effectively with demen-
        tia disorders (e.g., suppressing our dualistic biases). We need
        self-control when accepting or adjusting to another person's
        reality because it means overcoming our inherent egocentric
        perspective. Lieberman, *Social,* 208–16; Jessica R. Cohen,
        Elliot T. Berkman, and Matthew D. Lieberman, "Intentional
        and Incidental Self-Control in Ventrolateral PFC," *Principles of
        Frontal Lobe Function* 2 (2013): 417–40; Charlotte E. Hart-
        wright, Ian A. Apperly, and Peter C. Hansen, "The Special Case
        of Self-Perspective Inhibition in Mental, but Not Non-Mental,
        Representation," *Neuropsychologia* 67 (2015): 183–92.

97   **unreasonable demands:** Disregarding unfairness activates
        self-control in the brain because humans (and other mammals)

have evolved to be very sensitive to fairness violations. Golnaz Tabibnia, Ajay B. Satpute, and Matthew D. Lieberman, "The Sunny Side of Fairness: Preference for Fairness Activates Reward Circuitry (and Disregarding Unfairness Activates Self-Control Circuitry)," *Psychological Science* 19.4 (2008): 339–47.

97 **"mental brakes":** Lieberman calls the rVLPFC region the brain's "braking system."

98 **a state of ego depletion:** Roy F. Baumeister et al., "Ego Depletion: Is the Active Self a Limited Resource?" in *Self-Regulation and Self-control* (Routledge, 2018), 16–44. A good review of ego depletion research can be found in Mark Muraven, Jacek Buczny, and Kyle F. Law, "Ego Depletion: Theory and Evidence," (2019). For an overview of criticism and defense of the concept of ego depletion, see Malte Friese et al., "Is Ego Depletion Real? An Analysis of Arguments," *Personality and Social Psychology Review* 23.2 (2019): 107–31.

98 **we should rid ourselves of this "absolutist" approach:** Patricia S. Churchland, *Brain-wise: Studies in Neurophilosophy* (MIT Press, 2002), 214–18.

99 **optimal ranges of decision-making:** Patricia S. Churchland, "Neuroscience, Choice and Responsibility," *Topics in Integrative Neuroscience* (2008): 1.

99 **A protein called leptin:** Churchland was alluding to the article "Fat and Free Will," *Nature Neuroscience* 3, no. 11 (November 1, 2000): 1057. For recent research on leptin's critical role in obesity-related complications, see Olof S. Dallner et al., "Dysregulation of a Long Noncoding RNA Reduces Leptin Leading to a Leptin-Responsive Form of Obesity," *Nature Medicine* 25.3 (2019): 507–16, and Milan Obradovic et al., "Leptin and Obesity: Role and Clinical Implication," *Frontiers in Endocrinology* 12 (2021): 585887. On other genetic vulnerability for obesity, see Ruth J. F. Loos and Giles S. H. Yeo, "The Genetics of Obesity: From Discovery to Biology," *Nature Reviews Genetics* 23.2 (2022): 120–33.

7 My Dinner with Stefan Zweig

101 **three French citizens:** Jean-Paul Sartre, *No Exit and Three Other Plays,* translated by Stuart Gilbert (Vintage, 1989).

106 **to disapprove of Garcin:** Sartre describes this "inauthenticity" as acting in bad faith by letting others define you. Jean-Paul Sartre, *Being and Nothingness,* translated by Hazel E. Barnes (Washington Square Press, 1993).

107 **is most likely a fiction:** To truly understand self-processing in the brain, Lieberman argues that it is essential to take social

perception and reasoning into account. Not only is the "self" something that is constantly being constructed by many parts of the brain, it is heavily affected by interpersonal influence. Matthew D. Lieberman and Jennifer H. Pfeifer, "The Self and Social Perception: Three Kinds of Questions in Social Cognitive Neuroscience," in *The Cognitive Neuroscience of Social Behaviour* (Psychology Press, 2004), 207–48.

107   **The medial prefrontal cortex (MPFC):** There is a great deal of neurological overlap between social reasoning and self-assessment. Kevin N. Ochsner et al., "The Neural Correlates of Direct and Reflected Self-Knowledge," *Neuroimage* 28.4 (2005): 797–814; Jennifer H. Pfeifer, Matthew D. Lieberman, and Mirella Dapretto, "'I Know You Are But What Am I?!': Neural Bases of Self- and Social Knowledge Retrieval in Children and Adults," *Journal of Cognitive Neuroscience* 19.8 (2007): 1323–37; Joseph M. Moran, William M. Kelley, and Todd F. Heatherton, "What Can the Organization of the Brain's Default Mode Network Tell Us About Self-Knowledge?" *Frontiers in Human Neuroscience* 7 (2013): 391; Adrianna C. Jenkins and Jason P. Mitchell, "Medial Prefrontal Cortex Subserves Diverse Forms of Self-Reflection," *Social Neuroscience* 6.3 (2011): 211–18.

107   **"a superhighway":** Lieberman, *Social,* 198.

107   **"evolution's sneakiest ploy":** Ibid., 189.

107   **whose brains naturally absorb the worldview of other brains:** Ibid., 194–202.

108   **The activity of the MPFC is a neural habit:** Marcus E. Raichle et al., "A Default Mode of Brain Function," *Proceedings of the National Academy of Sciences* 98.2 (2001): 676–82; Wei Gao et al., "Evidence on the Emergence of the Brain's Default Network from 2-Week-Old to 2-Year-Old Healthy Pediatric Subjects," *Proceedings of the National Academy of Sciences* 106.16 (2009): 6790–95.

108   **Evolution could have pushed us toward:** Lieberman, *Social,* 22–33. Some argue that the reason our brains became bigger is from the pressures of managing increasingly complex social structures. Our large brains, in other words, are there to help us navigate the social world. F. Javier Pérez-Barbería, Susanne Shultz, and Robin I. M. Dunbar, "Evidence for Coevolution of Sociality and Relative Brain Size in Three Orders of Mammals," *Evolution* 61.12 (2007): 2811–21.

109   **this interaction *is* the experiment:** Kipling D. Williams and Blair Jarvis, "Cyberball: A Program for Use in Research on Interpersonal Ostracism and Acceptance," *Behavior Research Methods* 38.1 (2006): 174–80; Kipling D. Williams, Christopher K. T. Cheung, and Wilma Choi, "Cyberostracism: Effects

of Being Ignored over the Internet," *Journal of Personality and Social Psychology* 79.5 (2000): 748.

109   **replicated the Cyberball experiment:** Naomi I. Eisenberger, Matthew D. Lieberman, and Kipling D. Williams, "Does Rejection Hurt? An fMRI Study of Social Exclusion," *Science* 302.5643 (2003): 290–92.

110   **Even after they knew it was a machine:** Lisa Zadro, Kipling D. Williams, and Rick Richardson, "How Low Can You Go? Ostracism by a Computer Is Sufficient to Lower Self-Reported Levels of Belonging, Control, Self-Esteem, and Meaningful Existence," *Journal of Experimental Social Psychology* 40.4 (2004): 560–67.

110   **Rejection literally hurts:** Naomi I. Eisenberger and Matthew D. Lieberman, "Why Rejection Hurts: A Common Neural Alarm System for Physical and Social Pain," *Trends in Cognitive Sciences* 8.7 (2004): 294–300.

110   **perhaps Tylenol can help:** C. Nathan DeWall et al., "Acetaminophen Reduces Social Pain: Behavioral and Neural Evidence," *Psychological Science* 21.7 (2010): 931–37.

110   **researchers instructed two groups to play Cyberball:** Naomi I. Eisenberger, "The Neural Bases of Social Pain: Evidence for Shared Representations with Physical Pain," *Psychosomatic Medicine* 74.2 (2012): 126.

111   **our attachment system piggybacks on our physical pain system:** Jaak Panksepp et al., "The Biology of Social Attachments: Opiates Alleviate Separation Distress," *Biological Psychiatry* 13.5 (1978): 607–18.; Eric E. Nelson and Jaak Panksepp, "Brain Substrates of Infant-Mother Attachment: Contributions of Opioids, Oxytocin, and Norepinephrine," *Neuroscience and Biobehavioral Reviews* 22.3 (1998): 437–52.

111   **an adaptive signal that urges us to keep close:** Geoff MacDonald and Mark R. Leary, "Why Does Social Exclusion Hurt? The Relationship Between Social and Physical Pain," *Psychological Bulletin* 131.2 (2005): 202.

111   **without the pain of separation and isolation:** Paul D. MacLean and John D. Newman, "Role of Midline Frontolimbic Cortex in Production of the Isolation Call of Squirrel Monkeys," *Brain Research* 450.1–2 (1988): 111–23; Bryan W. Robinson, "Vocalization Evoked from Forebrain in Macaca Mulatta," *Physiology and Behavior* 2.4 (1967): 345–54. From these studies, Lieberman logically concludes the importance of the dACC to mother-child attachment and thus to survival. Lieberman, *Social*, 55.

111   **in one unpleasant experiment:** John S. Stamm, "The Function of the Median Cerebral Cortex in Maternal Behavior of Rats," *Journal of Comparative and Physiological Psychology* 48.4 (1955): 347.

111–12 **to hone and practice our social reasoning skills:** Nicholas K. Humphrey, "Nature's Psychologists," *New Scientist* 1109 (1978): 900–904.

8   The Mastermind

113 **Damasio introduces us to an unusual patient:** Antonio Damasio, *Descartes' Error: Emotion, Reason, and the Human Brain* (Random House, 2006), 34–51.

116 **"crazy and catatonic" or "insane and idiotic":** The shame and stigma associated with dementia in Asian populations, among other minority groups (including Hispanics, African Americans, and Native Americans), has been shown to contribute to underdetection of the disease, delayed diagnosis, and general barriers to care and management. Sahnah Lim et al., "Alzheimer's Disease and Its Related Dementias Among Asian Americans, Native Hawaiians, and Pacific Islanders: A Scoping Review," *Journal of Alzheimer's Disease* 77.2 (2020): 523–37.

121 **he was inclined to see reason as something separate:** Damasio explains that he was so concerned with Elliot's intelligence and rationality that he just did not pay much attention to emotions. Damasio, *Descartes' Error*, 44.

121 **from Plato's time to the twenty-first century:** D. Keltner and J. S. Lerner, *Emotion*, in D. T. Gilbert, S. T. Fiske, and G. Lindzey, eds., *Handbook of Social Psychology* (2010).

122 **no such thing as "pure" reason:** Specifically, scholars of decision making want to get away from the dichotomy of hot and cold, reason versus emotion, and instead strive to understand reason as a function of multiple, overlapping modalities. Elizabeth A. Phelps, Karolina M. Lempert, and Peter Sokol-Hessner, "Emotion and Decision Making: Multiple Modulatory Neural Circuits," *Annual Review of Neuroscience* 37.1 (2014): 263–87; Gerald L. Clore, "Psychology and the Rationality of Emotion," *Modern Theology* 27.2 (2011): 325–38; Robert Oum and Debra Lieberman, "Emotion Is Cognition: An Information-Processing View of the Mind," in *Do Emotions Help or Hurt Decision Making? A Hedgefoxian Perspective* (Russell Sage Foundation, 2007), 133–54.

122 **The "low" or "downstairs" compartments:** Damasio, *Descartes' Error*, 128.

122 **"the cortical networks on which feelings rely":** Ibid., xvi.

122 **"somatic markers," and he argues that they are indispensable:** Antonio R. Damasio, "The Somatic Marker Hypothesis and the Possible Functions of the Prefrontal Cortex,"

Philosophical Transactions of the Royal Society of London. Series B: Biological Sciences 351.1346 (1996): 1413–20.

123 **our mind would have to sift through numerous options:** Emadeddin Rahmanian Koshkaki and Sepideh Solhi, "The Facilitating Role of Negative Emotion in Decision Making Process: A Hierarchy of Effects Model Approach," *Journal of High Technology Management Research* 27.2 (2016): 119–28; Norbert Schwarz, "Feelings as Information: Informational and Motivational Functions of Affective States," in E. T. Higgins and R. M. Sorrentino, eds., *Handbook of Motivation and Cognition: Foundations of Social Behavior,* vol. 2 (New York: Guilford Press, 1990), 527–61.

125 **This is called the *affect heuristic*:** For a good overview of what affect heuristics do, see Paul Slovic et al., "Rational Actors or Rational Fools: Implications of the Affect Heuristic for Behavioral Economics," *Journal of Socio-Economics* 31.4 (2002): 329–42. For more on how we tend to use feelings to determine how we think and decide, see Melissa L. Finucane et al., "The Affect Heuristic in Judgments of Risks and Benefits," *Journal of Behavioral Decision Making* 13.1 (2000): 1–17. For a general overview of the significant role of emotions in decision making, see Jennifer S. Lerner et al., "Emotion and Decision Making," *Annual Review of Psychology* 66.1 (2015).

127 **had to learn to "speak Alzheimer's":** I am alluding to the book *Learning to Speak Alzheimer's,* which teaches caregivers effective strategies for communicating with people suffering from dementia disorders. Joanne Koenig Coste, *Learning to Speak Alzheimer's: A Groundbreaking Approach for Everyone Dealing with the Disease* (Houghton Mifflin Harcourt, 2004).

130 **beliefs are intrinsically tied to feelings:** Gerald L. Clore and Karen Gasper, "Feeling Is Believing: Some Affective Influences on Belief," in N. H. Frijda, A.S.R. Manstead, and S. Bem, eds., *Emotions and Beliefs: How Do Emotions Influence Beliefs?* (Cambridge: Cambridge University Press, 2000), 10–44.

130 **believing, in fact, is automatic:** We are so wired to believe or accept things as fact that our mind even tries to make sense of nonsense. Daniel T. Gilbert, Douglas S. Krull, and Patrick S. Malone, "Unbelieving the Unbelievable: Some Problems in the Rejection of False Information," *Journal of Personality and Social Psychology* 59.4 (1990): 601.

130 **take what people say at face value:** For a good overview of our tendency to believe what people say, see Timothy R. Levine, "Truth-Default Theory (TDT): A Theory of Human Deception and Deception Detection," *Journal of Language and*

Social Psychology 33.4 (2014): 378–92. We are so prone to believing that we tend to believe insincere flattery not only from people, but also from mindless computers. Elaine Chan and Jaideep Sengupta, "Insincere Flattery Actually Works: A Dual Attitudes Perspective," *Journal of Marketing Research* 47.1 (2010): 122–33; Brian J. Fogg and Clifford Nass, "Silicon Sycophants: The Effects of Computers That Flatter," *International Journal of Human-Computer Studies* 46.5 (1997): 551–61.

9   Ah Humanity

133   **"Bartleby, the Scrivener":** Herman Melville, *Billy Budd, Sailor and Other Stories* (Signet Classics, 1961).

133   **"a motionless young man":** Melville, *Bartleby,* 110.

133   **"silently, palely, mechanically":** Ibid., 111.

133   **"touched and disconcerted me":** Ibid., 113.

134   **there has been no shortage of critics:** For a good review of who critics say Bartleby represents, see Milton R. Stern, "Towards 'Bartleby the Scrivener,'" *Bloom's Modern Critical Views: Herman Melville* (Chelsea House, 1979): 13–38.

136   **"fraternal melancholy":** Melville, *Bartleby,* 120.

136   **to make sense of people's behavior:** This chapter will explain why our minds are biologically predisposed to look for intentions, beliefs, and goals.

136   **sticks her tongue out at us:** Andrew N. Meltzoff and M. Keith Moore, "Newborn Infants Imitate Adult Facial Gestures," *Child Development* (1983): 702–709; Andrew N. Meltzoff and M. Keith Moore, "Imitation of Facial and Manual Gestures by Human Neonates," *Science* 198.4312 (1977): 75–78; Giuseppe Di Pellegrino et al., "Understanding Motor Events: A Neurophysiological Study," *Experimental Brain Research* 91.1 (1992): 176–80; Luciano Fadiga et al., "Motor Facilitation During Action Observation: A Magnetic Stimulation Study," *Journal of Neurophysiology* 73.6 (1995): 2608–11; G. Rizzolatti et al., "Localization of Cortical Areas Responsive to the Observation of Hand Grasping Movements in Humans: A PET Study," *Experimental Brain Research* 111.2 (1996): 246–52; Vittorio Gallese et al., "Action Recognition in the Premotor Cortex," *Brain* 119.2 (1996): 593–609.

136   **"mirror neurons":** Giacomo Rizzolatti and Maddalena Fabbri-Destro, "Mirror Neurons," *Scholarpedia* 3.1 (2008): 2055; Maddalena Fabbri-Destro and Giacomo Rizzolatti, "Mirror Neurons and Mirror Systems in Monkeys and Humans," *Physiology* 23.3 (2008): 171–79; Flavia Filimon et al.,

"Human Cortical Representations for Reaching: Mirror Neurons for Execution, Observation, and Imagery," *Neuroimage* 37.4 (2007): 1315–28.

136 **The mirroring impulse or "mimicry system":** Giacomo Rizzolatti and Maddalena Fabbri-Destro, "The Mirror System and Its Role in Social Cognition," *Current Opinion in Neurobiology* 18.2 (2008): 179–84; Marco Iacoboni et al., "Grasping the Intentions of Others with One's Own Mirror Neuron System," *PLoS Biology* 3.3 (2005): e79.

136–37 **We literally feel other people's pain:** We vicariously feel both physical and emotional pain. Of course, observing pain and experiencing it is not a one-to-one experience in the brain; there is a great deal of shared neural representation. Philip L. Jackson, Andrew N. Meltzoff, and Jean Decety, "How Do We Perceive the Pain of Others? A Window into the Neural Processes Involved in Empathy," *Neuroimage* 24.3 (2005): 771–79; Claus Lamm, Jean Decety, and Tania Singer, "Meta-analytic Evidence for Common and Distinct Neural Networks Associated with Directly Experienced Pain and Empathy for Pain," *Neuroimage* 54.3 (2011): 2492–2502; Claus Lamm et al., "What Are You Feeling? Using Functional Magnetic Resonance Imaging to Assess the Modulation of Sensory and Affective Responses During Empathy for Pain," *PloS One* 2.12 (2007): e1292; Kevin N. Ochsner et al., "Your Pain or Mine? Common and Distinct Neural Systems Supporting the Perception of Pain in Self and Other," *Social Cognitive and Affective Neuroscience* 3.2 (2008): 144–60; Sören Krach et al., "Your Flaws Are My Pain: Linking Empathy to Vicarious Embarrassment," *PloS One* 6.4 (2011): e18675; Bruno Wicker et al., "Both of Us Disgusted in My Insula: The Common Neural Basis of Seeing and Feeling Disgust," *Neuron* 40.3 (2003): 655–64; Matthew Botvinick et al., "Viewing Facial Expressions of Pain Engages Cortical Areas Involved in the Direct Experience of Pain," *Neuroimage* 25.1 (2005): 312–19.

137 **busily copying the reactions of others:** Ulf Dimberg, "Facial Reactions to Facial Expressions," *Psychophysiology* 19.6 (1982): 643–47; Ulf Dimberg and Monika Thunberg, "Rapid Facial Reactions to Emotional Facial Expressions," *Scandinavian Journal of Psychology* 39.1 (1998): 39–45; Ulf Dimberg, Monika Thunberg, and Kurt Elmehed, "Unconscious Facial Reactions to Emotional Facial Expressions," *Psychological Science* 11.1 (2000): 86–89; Lars-Olov Lundqvist and Ulf Dimberg, "Facial Expressions Are Contagious," *Journal of Psychophysiology* 9 (1995): 203–11; Krystyna Rymarczyk et al., "Empathy in Facial Mimicry of Fear and Disgust: Simultaneous

EMG-fMRI Recordings During Observation of Static and Dynamic Facial Expressions," *Frontiers in Psychology* 10 (2019): 701.

137 **(Tellingly, people injected with Botox):** David A. Havas et al., "Cosmetic Use of Botulinum Toxin-A Affects Processing of Emotional Language," *Psychological Science* 21.7 (2010): 895–900. If something inhibits our ability to make facial expressions, we become less capable of experiencing other people's emotions, because imitating others' expressions is one way we understand how others feel. Paula M. Niedenthal et al., "When Did Her Smile Drop? Facial Mimicry and the Influences of Emotional State on the Detection of Change in Emotional Expression," *Cognition and Emotion* 15.6 (2001): 853–64; David T. Neal and Tanya L. Chartrand, "Embodied Emotion Perception: Amplifying and Dampening Facial Feedback Modulates Emotion Perception Accuracy," *Social Psychological and Personality Science* 2.6 (2011): 673–78.

137 **if we take a painkiller:** Dominik Mischkowski, Jennifer Crocker, and Baldwin M. Way. "From Painkiller to Empathy Killer: Acetaminophen (Paracetamol) Reduces Empathy for Pain," *Social Cognitive and Affective Neuroscience* 11.9 (2016): 1345–53.

137 **"emotional contagion":** Elaine Hatfield, John T. Cacioppo, and Richard L. Rapson, "Emotional Contagion," *Studies in Emotion and Social Interaction* (Cambridge University Press, 1994); Elaine Hatfield et al., "New Perspectives on Emotional Contagion: A Review of Classic and Recent Research on Facial Mimicry and Contagion," *Interpersona: An International Journal on Personal Relationships* 8.2 (2014).

137 **a by-product of our mimicry system:** Stephanie D. Preston and Frans B. M. de Waal, "Empathy: Its Ultimate and Proximate Bases," *Behavioral and Brain Sciences* 25.1 (2002): 1–20; Hanna Drimalla et al., "From Face to Face: The Contribution of Facial Mimicry to Cognitive and Emotional Empathy," *Cognition and Emotion* 33.8 (2019): 1672–86; Jean Decety and Philip L. Jackson, "A Social-Neuroscience Perspective on Empathy," *Current Directions in Psychological Science* 15.2 (2006): 54–58; Shinya Yamamoto, "Primate Empathy: Three Factors and Their Combinations for Empathy-Related Phenomena," *Wiley Interdisciplinary Reviews: Cognitive Science* 8.3 (2017): e1431; Frans B. M. de Waal, "The Antiquity of Empathy," *Science* 336.6083 (2012): 874–76; Lian T. Rameson and Matthew D. Lieberman, "Empathy: A Social Cognitive Neuroscience Approach," *Social and Personality Psychology Compass* 3.1 (2009): 94–110. It should be noted that the mimicry system is considered just one path to empathy.

137 **as the psychologist Paul Bloom notes:** Paul Bloom, *Against Empathy: The Case for Rational Compassion* (Ecco, 2016), 65–67. In fact, putting yourself in other people's shoes actually decreases accuracy. Nicholas Epley, *Mindwise: Why We Misunderstand What Others Think, Believe, Feel, and Want* (Vintage, 2015), 168–69; Nicholas Epley, Eugene M. Caruso, and Max H. Bazerman, "When Perspective Taking Increases Taking: Reactive Egoism in Social Interaction," *Journal of Personality and Social Psychology* 91.5 (2006): 872. Because imagining what it's like to have dementia disorders might lead to egocentric error, the best way to mitigate this error is simply to ask people questions directly about their state of mind. Epley, *Mindwise*, 173. This is of course complicated when the person is in a late stage of a dementia disorder. Not knowing the patient's state of mind is one of the great challenges of caregiving and has many caregivers projecting their emotions onto the patient.

138 **Psychologists call this "mind reading":** David Premack and Guy Woodruff, "Does the Chimpanzee Have a Theory of Mind?" *Behavioral and Brain Sciences* 1.4 (1978): 515–26; Helen L. Gallagher and Christopher D. Frith, "Functional Imaging of 'Theory of Mind,'" *Trends in Cognitive Sciences* 7.2 (2003): 77–83; James K. Rilling et al., "The Neural Correlates of Theory of Mind Within Interpersonal Interactions," *Neuroimage* 22.4 (2004): 1694–1703; David M. Amodio and Chris D. Frith (2006), "Meeting of Minds: The Medial Frontal Cortex and Social Cognition," in *Discovering the Social Mind: Selected Works of Christopher D. Frith* (Psychology Press, 2016), 183–207.

138 **In the elegant Heider-Simmel triangle experiment:** Fritz Heider and Marianne Simmel, "An Experimental Study of Apparent Behavior," *American Journal of Psychology* 57.2 (1944): 243–59.

138 **when scientists could perform an MRI of the brain:** Fulvia Castelli et al., "Movement and Mind: A Functional Imaging Study of Perception and Interpretation of Complex Intentional Movement Patterns," *Social Neuroscience: Key Readings* (2005): 155; Fulvia Castelli et al., "Movement and Mind: A Functional Imaging Study of Perception and Interpretation of Complex Intentional Movement Patterns," in *Social Neuroscience* (Psychology Press, 2013), 155–69.

138 **our brain's greatest evolutionary aspiration:** For an overview of the importance of prediction, see Andy Clark, "Whatever Next? Predictive Brains, Situated Agents, and the Future of Cognitive Science," *Behavioral and Brain Sciences* 36.3 (2013): 181–204.

139 **to see others as willful rather than mindless:** Elliot C. Brown and Martin Brüne, "The Role of Prediction in Social Neuroscience," *Frontiers in Human Neuroscience* 6 (2012): 147.

139 **"intentional stance":** Daniel Clement Dennett, *The Intentional Stance* (MIT Press, 1987). The concept of the "intentional stance" has been supported in studies of social neuroscience. Bryan T. Denny et al., "A Meta-analysis of Functional Neuroimaging Studies of Self- and Other Judgments Reveals a Spatial Gradient for Mentalizing in Medial Prefrontal Cortex," *Journal of Cognitive Neuroscience* 24.8 (2012): 1742–52; Rogier B. Mars et al., "On the Relationship Between the 'Default Mode Network' and the 'Social Brain,'" *Frontiers in Human Neuroscience* 6 (2012): 189; Robert P. Spunt, Meghan L. Meyer, and Matthew D. Lieberman, "The Default Mode of Human Brain Function Primes the Intentional Stance," *Journal of Cognitive Neuroscience* 27.6 (2015): 1116–24.

139 **things that exhibit preferences and intentions:** Nicholas Epley, Adam Waytz, and John T. Cacioppo, "On Seeing Human: A Three-Factor Theory of Anthropomorphism," *Psychological Review* 114.4 (2007): 864; Adam Waytz et al., "Making Sense by Making Sentient: Effectance Motivation Increases Anthropomorphism," *Journal of Personality and Social Psychology* 99.3 (2010): 410.

139 **"innate and incurable disorder":** Melville, *Bartleby,* 122.

140 **the farther we're removed from others:** Epley, *Mindwise,* 43, 49; Min Kyung Lee, Nathaniel Fruchter, and Laura Dabbish, "Making Decisions from a Distance: The Impact of Technological Mediation on Riskiness and Dehumanization," *CSCW '15: Proceedings of the 18th ACM Conference on Computer Supported Cooperative Work & Social Computing,* Human-Computer Interaction Institute, Heinz College, Carnegie Mellon University, 2015, 1576–89.

141 **cause us to see the physical world differently:** Lieberman, *Social,* 186.

141 **We are, after all, dualistic creatures:** See chapter 5.

141 **We perceive the physical world as abiding by preordained laws:** Daniel C. Dennett, *Kinds of Minds: Toward an Understanding of Consciousness* (Basic Books, 1996), 27–36.

141 **When we no longer perceive intention:** As established, an activated MPFC means we are thinking of others and thus engaged in social reasoning. Amodio and Frith, "Meeting of Minds." When less engaged, our mind tends to see these people as "out-groups." Lasana T. Harris and Susan T. Fiske, "Social Groups That Elicit Disgust Are Differentially Processed in mPFC," *Social Cognitive and Affective Neuroscience* 2.1

(2007): 45–51; Lasana T. Harris and Susan T. Fiske, "Dehumanizing the Lowest of the Low: Neuroimaging Responses to Extreme Out-Groups," *Psychological Science* 17.10 (2006): 847–53; Susan T. Fiske, "From Dehumanization and Objectification to Rehumanization: Neuroimaging Studies on the Building Blocks of Empathy," *Annals of the New York Academy of Sciences* 1167.1 (2009): 31–34.

141   **the neurological expression of "dehumanization":** Lasana T. Harris and Susan T. Fiske, "Perceiving Humanity or Not: A Social Neuroscience Approach to Dehumanized Perception," *Social Neuroscience: Toward Understanding the Underpinnings of the Social Mind* (2011): 123–34; Celia Guillard and Lasana T. Harris, "The Neuroscience of Dehumanization and Its Implications for Political Violence," in *Propaganda and International Criminal Law* (Routledge, 2019), 199–216.

142   **"Ah Bartleby! Ah humanity":** Melville, *Bartleby*, 140.

142   **people attribute more "human" qualities to themselves:** Nick Haslam et al., "More Human than You: Attributing Humanness to Self and Others," *Journal of Personality and Social Psychology* 89.6 (2005): 937.

142   **Empathy thus is accorded more to those we identify with:** The more different we find other people from ourselves, the less empathy we have for them. Shihui Han, "Neurocognitive Basis of Racial Ingroup Bias in Empathy," *Trends in Cognitive Sciences* 22.5 (2018): 400–421. One of those qualities that we feel makes us "human" or gives minds value is free will. Not surprisingly, people believe they have more free will than others. Epley, *Mindwise*, 50–51; Emily Pronin and Matthew B. Kugler, "People Believe They Have More Free Will than Others," *Proceedings of the National Academy of Sciences* 107.52 (2010): 22469–74.

10   When the Right Thing Is the Wrong Thing

147   **a classic thought experiment:** Judith Jarvis Thomson, *Rights, Restitution, and Risk: Essays in Moral Theory* (Cambridge, Mass.: Harvard University Press, 1986).

148   **In one such experiment:** Joshua D. Greene et al., "An fMRI Investigation of Emotional Engagement in Moral Judgment," *Science* 293.5537 (2001): 2105–2108.

148   **Kant, who believed:** J. Greene, "The Secret Joke of Kant's Soul," in Walter Sinnott-Armstrong, ed., *Moral Psychology*, vol. 3, *The Neuroscience of Morality: Emotion, Disease, and Development* (MIT Press, 2007), 35–79.

148   **they are also essential in moral decision-making:** For a good review of the subject, see Joshua Greene and Jonathan

Haidt, "How (and Where) Does Moral Judgment Work?" *Trends in Cognitive Sciences* 6.12 (2002): 517–23; Jesse Prinz, "Sentimentalism and the Moral Brain," *Moral Brains: The Neuroscience of Morality* (2016): 45–73.

148 **a "social intuitionist" model:** Jonathan Haidt, "The Emotional Dog and Its Rational Tail: A Social Intuitionist Approach to Moral Judgment," *Psychological Review* 108.4 (2001): 814.

149 **the most advanced stage in human development:** Lawrence Kohlberg, "Stage and Sequence: The Cognitive-Developmental Approach to Socialization," *Handbook of Socialization Theory and Research* 347 (1969): 480. Kohlberg's cognitive-centered approach was heavily influenced by the work of Jean Piaget, who is still regarded as the most prominent developmental psychologist of the twentieth century. Jean Piaget, *The Moral Judgement of the Child,* translated by M. Gabain (Harmondsworth: Penguin, 1977), originally published 1932.

149 **"The emotions are . . . in charge of the temple of morality":** Jonathan Haidt, "The Moral Emotions," in R. J. Davidson, K. R. Scherer, and H. H. Goldsmith, eds., *Handbook of Affective Sciences* (Oxford University Press, 2003), 852.

149 **takes a "bottom-up" approach to the subject:** Frans de Waal and Stephen A. Sherblom, "Bottom-up Morality: The Basis of Human Morality in Our Primate Nature," *Journal of Moral Education* 47.2 (2018): 248–58.

149 **favor cooperation and exhibit a proclivity for fairness:** Sarah F. Brosnan and Frans de Waal, "Monkeys Reject Unequal Pay," *Nature* 425.6955 (2003): 297–99; Jessica C. Flack and Frans B. M. de Waal, "'Any Animal Whatever': Darwinian Building Blocks of Morality in Monkeys and Apes," *Journal of Consciousness Studies* 7.1–2 (2000): 1–29; Colt Halter, "Empathy and Fairness in Nonhuman Primates: Evolutionary Bases of Human Morality," *Intuition: The BYU Undergraduate Journal of Psychology* 14.2 (2019): 9.

149 **engage in complex interactions:** Marc Bekoff and Jessica Pierce, "Wild Justice: Honor and Fairness Among Beasts at Play," *American Journal of Play* 1.4 (2009): 451–75.

149–50 **the degree to which emotion or cognition comes into play:** Joshua D. Greene, "Dual-Process Morality and the Personal/Impersonal Distinction: A Reply to McGuire, Langdon, Coltheart, and Mackenzie," *Journal of Experimental Social Psychology* 45.3 (2009): 581–84.

151 **accepting a moral violation like unfairness:** Each time we resist the impulse to disapprove of a moral violation, it activates the dorsolateral prefrontal cortex (DLPFC), the part of our brain that's responsible for self-control. Aversion to moral

violations is automatic. Joshua D. Greene, "Why Are VMPFC Patients More Utilitarian? A Dual-Process Theory of Moral Judgment Explains," *Trends in Cognitive Sciences* 11.8 (2007): 322–23. As we saw in chapter 6, disregarding unfair treatment also activates self-control. Golnaz Tabibnia, Ajay B. Satpute, and Matthew D. Lieberman, "The Sunny Side of Fairness: Preference for Fairness Activates Reward Circuitry (and Disregarding Unfairness Activates Self-Control Circuitry)," *Psychological Science* 19.4 (2008): 339–47.

151 **to see intention in morally problematic behavior:** Specifically, people are more likely to think morally charged behavior is intentional if it has harmful effects. Joshua Knobe, "The Concept of Intentional Action: A Case Study in the Uses of Folk Psychology," *Philosophical Studies* 130.2 (2006): 203–31; Arudra Burra and Joshua Knobe, "The Folk Concepts of Intention and Intentional Action: A Cross-Cultural Study," *Journal of Cognition and Culture* 6.1–2 (2006): 113–32; Joshua Knobe and Gabriel S. Mendlow, "The Good, the Bad and the Blameworthy: Understanding the Role of Evaluative Reasoning in Folk Psychology," *Journal of Theoretical and Philosophical Psychology* 24.2 (2004): 252; Joshua Knobe, "Theory of Mind and Moral Cognition: Exploring the Connections," *Trends in Cognitive Sciences* 9.8 (2005): 357–59.

151 **"incompatibilist" position:** For an in-depth review of incompatibilism and compatibilism, see Paolo Galeazzi and Rasmus K. Rendsvig, "On the Foundations of the Problem of Free Will," *Episteme* (2022): 1–19.

151–52 **dementia disorders do not necessarily create a deterministic world:** The philosopher Joshua Knobe agrees that while dementia disorders are obviously not a straightforward case of determinism, it is still appropriate to apply the theory to dementia disorders.

152 **two hypothetical scenarios:** Shaun Nichols and Joshua Knobe, "Moral Responsibility and Determinism: The Cognitive Science of Folk Intuitions," *Nous* 41.4 (2007): 663–85. Again, Knobe agreed that even though dementia disorders don't directly align with the deterministic scenarios that he and Shaun Nichols created, he affirmed that the parallel that I drew from the reaction to his imaginary concrete and abstract situations and the real-life reactions that took place in my group is meaningful. Both affirm the role of emotion in our moral judgment.

153 **will most likely not influence our moral views:** Adina Roskies, "Neuroscientific Challenges to Free Will and Responsibility," *Trends in Cognitive Sciences* 10.9 (2006): 419–23;

Adina Roskies and Eddy Nahmias, "'Local Determination,' Even If We Could Find It, Does Not Challenge Free Will: Commentary on Marcelo Fischborn," *Philosophical Psychology* 30.1–2 (2017): 185–97.

153   **it dwells between people, between minds:** Michael Gazzaniga, *The Ethical Brain: The Science of Our Moral Dilemmas* (Ecco, 2006), 101–102.

154   **propaganda is used to invalidate:** Bloom, *Descartes' Baby,* 177.

154   **thereby eliciting disgust:** Feeling disgust and revulsion toward others predicts our likelihood to dehumanize them. Simone Schnall et al., "Disgust as Embodied Moral Judgment," *Personality and Social Psychology Bulletin* 34.8 (2008): 1096–1109; Erin E. Buckels and Paul D. Trapnell, "Disgust Facilitates Outgroup Dehumanization," *Group Processes and Intergroup Relations* 16.6 (2013): 771–80; Gordon Hodson, Nour Kteily, and Mark Hoffarth, "Of Filthy Pigs and Subhuman Mongrels: Dehumanization, Disgust, and Intergroup Prejudice," *TPM: Testing, Psychometrics, Methodology in Applied Psychology* 21.3 (2014); Allison L. Skinner and Caitlin M. Hudac, "'Yuck, You Disgust Me!' Affective Bias Against Interracial Couples," *Journal of Experimental Social Psychology* 68 (2017): 68–77. For evolutionary theory as to why disgust leads to dehumanization, see Alexander P. Landry, Elliott Ihm, and Jonathan W. Schooler, "Filthy Animals: Integrating the Behavioral Immune System and Disgust into a Model of Prophylactic Dehumanization," *Evolutionary Psychological Science* 8.2 (2022): 120–33. Recently, other emotions like anger and fear have been implicated in dehumanization. Roger Giner-Sorolla and Pascale Sophie Russell, "Not Just Disgust: Fear and Anger Also Relate to Intergroup Dehumanization," *Collabra: Psychology* 5.1 (2019). All this research underscores how deeply linked our moral prejudices are with our emotions.

154   **of reaffirming her moral standing:** Dennett explains that only "mind-havers" are guaranteed moral standing, which means you owe them and they owe you moral consideration. Dennett, *Kinds of Minds,* 4.

154   **have a "good" deep-down self:** It seems we even feel that our adversaries are fundamentally good. Julian De Freitas and Mina Cikara, "Deep Down My Enemy Is Good: Thinking About the True Self Reduces Intergroup Bias," *Journal of Experimental Social Psychology* 74 (2018): 307–16.

156   **"withdrawing [his] moral status":** Gazzaniga, *Ethical Brain,* 32.

11 Word Girl

171 **to be studied in isolation:** Simon Garrod and Martin J. Pickering, "Why Is Conversation So Easy?" *Trends in Cognitive Sciences* 8.1 (2004): 8–11.

171 **in which "interactive alignment" creates:** Simon Garrod and Martin J. Pickering, "Joint Action, Interactive Alignment, and Dialog," *Topics in Cognitive Science* 1.2 (2009): 292–304; Laura Menenti, Martin J. Pickering, and Simon C. Garrod, "Toward a Neural Basis of Interactive Alignment in Conversation," *Frontiers in Human Neuroscience* 6 (2012): 185.

171 **in the auditory or motor regions of the brain:** Greg J. Stephens, Lauren J. Silbert, and Uri Hasson, "Speaker–Listener Neural Coupling Underlies Successful Communication," *Proceedings of the National Academy of Sciences* 107.32 (2010): 14425–30.

171–72 **requiring neither deliberation nor conscious control:** Garrod and Pickering, "Why Is Conversation So Easy?"

172 **guided by our companion's speech:** Martin J. Pickering and Simon Garrod, "An Integrated Theory of Language Production and Comprehension." *Behavioral and Brain Sciences* 36.4 (2013): 329–47; Holly P. Branigan et al., "Syntactic Alignment and Participant Role in Dialogue," *Cognition* 104.2 (2007): 163–97; Susan E. Brennan and Herbert H. Clark, "Conceptual Pacts and Lexical Choice in Conversation," *Journal of Experimental Psychology: Learning, Memory, and Cognition* 22.6 (1996): 1482; Kevin Shockley, Marie-Vee Santana, and Carol A. Fowler, "Mutual Interpersonal Postural Constraints Are Involved In Cooperative Conversation," *Journal of Experimental Psychology: Human Perception and Performance* 29.2 (2003): 326.

173 **our minds try to imitate other minds:** Martin J. Pickering and Simon Garrod, "Do People Use Language Production to Make Predictions During Comprehension?" *Trends in Cognitive Sciences* 11.3 (2007): 105–10.

174 **"The lightning flashed":** Here Nietzsche touches on how "the popular mind" is primed to impose intentions even on mindless phenomena and how language reinforces this tendency. In a way, he anticipated work done by experimental philosophers on the subject of "folk psychology," which is a study of our mind's intuitions. Friedrich Nietzsche, *"On the Genealogy of Morals" and "Ecce Homo,"* translated by Walter Kaufmann (Vintage, 1967), 45.

174 **language inadvertently confirms:** Patrick Haggard, "Human Volition: Towards a Neuroscience of Will," *Nature Reviews Neuroscience* 9.12 (2008): 934–46.

177 **"This is becoming really insignificant":** Samuel Beckett, *I Can't Go On, I'll Go On: A Selection from Samuel Beckett's Work* (Grove Press, 1976), 443.

178 **"As long as we have faith in grammar":** Friedrich Nietzsche, "Twilight of the Idols," translated by Walter Kaufman, in *The Portable Nietzsche* (Penguin Books, 1976), 483.

178 **When communicating, we partially redress:** Dennett explains that words are powerful because they are inherently "resolvers of doubt and ambiguity," giving the impression of clarity. Dennett, *Kinds of Minds*, 8.

178 **as long as we converse, we can hope:** Another reason that conversation is inherently hopeful is that speakers tend to overestimate their effectiveness. Boaz Keysar and Anne S. Henly, "Speakers' Overestimation of Their Effectiveness," *Psychological Science* 13.3 (2002): 207–12; Becky Ka Ying Lau et al., "The Extreme Illusion of Understanding," *Journal of Experimental Psychology: General* (2022), advance online publication, doi.org/10.1037/xge0001213.

Epilogue

184 **what make the mind a marvel:** Daniel Kahneman, "The Marvels and the Flaws of Intuitive Thinking," in *The New Science of Decision-Making, Problem-Solving, and Prediction* (HarperCollins, 2013).

Index

About the Author

DASHA KIPER is the consulting clinical director of
support groups at an Alzheimer's organization and
has an MA in clinical psychology from Columbia
University. She has worked with both dementia
patients and caregivers.